LOVING
SOLUTIONS

OVERCOMING BARRIERS IN YOUR MARRIAGE

LOVING SOLUTIONS

OVERCOMING BARRIERS IN YOUR MARRIAGE

GARY CHAPMAN

AUTHOR OF THE FIVE LOVE LANGUAGES

NORTHFIELD PUBLISHING
CHICAGO

ISBN: 1-8812-73-91-1

3 5 7 9 10 8 6 4

Printed in the United States of America

To the many couples
who have shared their marital struggles with me,
and who have given me the extreme joy
of seeing them take the road to
reality living

TABLE OF CONTENTS

ACKNOWLEDGEMENTS

I am deeply indebted to the couples who have allowed me to be a part of their journey toward loving solutions in their marriages. For some, the journey has been extremely long and painful. For others, solutions came easier and earlier. For all, it has been a road of growth and discovery. I am privileged to have walked the road with them, and now to tell their stories. To them, this book is dedicated.

My appreciation to Tricia Kube, my administrative assistant for more than fifteen years; Tricia not only computerized the manuscript but offered many helpful suggestions. Jim Vincent, general editor at Northfield Publishing, was of immense help in polishing the final manuscript.

As always, I want to express my love and appreciation for Karolyn, my wife for more than thirty-five years. Together we have found our own "loving solutions." Her joyful spirit is a constant source of encouragement to me.

INTRODUCTION

I was in a Chicago suburb one cold Saturday morning, leading my Toward a Growing Marriage seminar, when I first met Maria. Earlier I had given the audience a summary of my book *Hope for the Separated: Wounded Marriages Can Be Healed*. I had encouraged audience members to get a copy for any of their friends who were separated. Maria had purchased the book and was holding it in her hands.

"Dr. Chapman, when are you going to write a book for me?" she asked.

"What do you mean?"

"I'm sure this book is good for those who are already separated," she said, "but what about people like me? My husband and I are not separated. We have been married for seventeen years. Neither of us believe in divorce; we have strong religious convictions, but our marriage is miserable. We have some really big problems that we have never been able to resolve. We'll fight about them and then make up, and things will be fine for a few weeks. Then we're back into warfare again. We need help."

"We went for counseling one time for a few sessions, but it didn't seem to help. We've read some books on marriage, but they just don't seem to deal with our problems. I know there must be other couples like us who really want their marriage to work but haven't been able to find answers."

I found out later that Maria was living with an alcoholic husband who for that and other reasons was also irresponsible in his work patterns. Thus, finances had been a problem all their marriage.

Since my conversation with Maria, I have written three more books, but I have never forgotten Maria's question, "When are you going to write a book for me?" I have had no further contact with Maria and do not know what has happened in her marriage. But if I could see her again, I would say "Maria, this one's for you." Yes, for Maria—and thousands of others like her who sincerely want to make their marriage work but have not yet found solutions to major problems.

Three factors motivated me to write this book. First, large numbers of people like Maria have approached me at my seminars, asking for practical help with what I and they consider to be major barriers to marital unity, the kind of issues that we do not have time to deal with in a weekend seminar—problems that have lingered for years and whose roots run deep; problems that, if they are not solved, can and do destroy many marriages.

The second catalyst for writing this book is the memory of my own struggles in the early years of my marriage. I well remember the pain that followed months of trying to do what I thought was right, yet to no avail. I remember the sense of helplessness that overwhelmed me, the recurring thought that I was married to someone with whom I would never have real intimacy. The problems seemed so deep and my resources so shallow that I found it difficult even to pursue "another approach." But there were answers and eventually, we found them. Karolyn and I have been married for more than thirty-five years now and have come to experience an intimacy I never dreamed possible. The pain is a distant memory, but it motivates me to seek to help others who struggle as sincerely as we.

The third force that pushes me to write this book is the steady stream of individuals with whom I have worked in the counseling office over the past twenty-five years, people who have had to deal with alcoholism, verbal and physical abuse, the unfaithfulness of a spouse, a controlling personality; or those who have had to deal with a painful past involving child abuse or low self-esteem; and some who have been married to workaholics and others to irresponsible mates. One of the rewards of counseling is seeing these kinds of people take responsible steps to deal with genuine problems, to support them in their efforts, and to see the fruit of improved relationships. I am convinced that their successes need a wider audience and that perhaps the steps they took will also give guidance to others.

I will change their names and enough details to protect their privacy, but the accounts you will read in the following pages depict the lives of real people with real problems who found meaningful solutions.

In each chapter, I will seek to identify first of all the nature of the specific problem and draw from social and psychological research where available. In questions of morality, I will offer guidelines from my own Judeo-Christian heritage. My intended purpose is to give practical suggestions on how to move your marriage from where it is to where you want it to be. Obviously I cannot guarantee success, but I can guarantee the satisfaction of knowing that you have given your marriage your best efforts. It is my sincere desire that this book will help channel your efforts into more productive methods.

Yes, Maria, this one's for you.

THE CRIES FOR SOLUTIONS

$\mathcal{B}$etsy was a beautiful young lady from a fine Southern home. Her parents were pillars in the community, and her life was a picture of success. At least, that was the way it appeared. But in my office, her beautiful face was streaked with rivulets of tears.

"We've been married for six years," she said. "Everyone thinks that we have a perfect marriage. The fact is, my husband and I have never been sexually intimate in the six years of our marriage and what hurts me the most is that it doesn't seem to matter to him. I read books that talk about the male sex drive, but I don't see it in my husband. He seems to have no interest at all. For awhile, it didn't bother me because I thought it would change, but now I don't think it will.

"I want to have intimacy in my marriage and I don't want to leave my husband, but I don't know what to do. We've talked about it a few times and he's told me not to worry about it, but I do worry about it. It's just not right; something is wrong and I don't know what to do about it." Living with unmet sexual needs can lead to intense feelings of rejection.

Betsy is not alone in her marital struggles. Although their symptoms may be different from Betsy's, thousands of couples are struggling in their marriages. They could write a book entitled *How To Be Married and Miserable.* Some of them have been married five years and others twenty-five years. They entered marriage with the same high hopes with which most of us said "I do." They never intended to be miserable; in fact, they dreamed that in marriage they would be supremely happy. Some of them were happy before they got married and anticipated that marriage would simply enhance their already exciting life. Others entered marriage with a deeply dysfunctional history. Their hope was that in marriage, they would finally discover meaning and happiness. In every case, the man and woman anticipated that marriage would be a road leading upward, that whatever life had been to that point, it would get better after marriage.

THE ROAD DOWNWARD

Their experience, though, has been that since the mountain-top celebration of the wedding, the road has been winding steadily downward. There have been a few peaks of enjoyment and a few curves that offered a promising vista. But the vista later turned out to be a mirage; and the marital road again turned downward. For a long time, they have lived in the valley of pain, emptiness, and frustration.

Many such couples have already opted for divorce. They saw it as the only exit from a lifetime of misery. Some chose divorce simply as a survival technique. Most chose it with a sincere desire that life would get better somewhere, sometime, with someone. Thousands of other couples are considering divorce as the solution; perhaps you or someone you know is. We will examine the merits of the divorce decision in the next chapter. At this point, let me just note that very few seekers have found greater happiness in another marriage or in remaining single. Many have found a second marriage to be a repeat performance of the first, the major difference being that they reached the valley of despair sooner the second time around.

There is another host of couples who have remained married

but who feel miserable. They really don't want to divorce. For many of them, their religious beliefs discourage them from taking that exit. Others are strongly motivated to keep their marriage together for the children, while others are finding enough moments of happiness or support to keep their hopes for a better marriage alive.

These husbands and wives sincerely hope that things will get better. Many feel that they have tried to deal with the issues that have kept them from marital unity. Most are discouraged with the results. If they have gone for counseling, it has not been very productive. If they have read books, they have read them alone wishing that their spouse could hear what the distant author is saying and be moved to change. Some have tried the calm, cool, straightforward method of gentle confrontation. They have been met with a silent audience and no response. Some in desperation have tried yelling and screaming. Their pain has been so intense that they have actually lost control in trying to express it. Their loud cry for help has been met, in some cases, with a counterattack and in others by withdrawal.

The problems with which these married couples grapple are not little issues. They cannot be solved by quiet parlor talk. Nor do the problems melt under the intense heat of pious platitudes. The problems are like cancer eating away at the vitality of the marriage. The problems vary from couple to couple, but the intensity of the pain runs deep for all. Let me take you behind closed doors into the privacy of my counseling office and let you listen as husbands and wives share "their situation." Let me also invite you to join me "on the road" as I lead marriage seminars across the country. Listen to what people tell me before and after our sessions. For most, I am not the first to hear their tale of pain. Hopefully, listening to their cries will give you an idea of the kind of problems we will be dealing with in this book.

STORIES FROM THE FRONT

I met Raphael in beautiful sunny southern California. He was the picture of health, and I supposed that his bronze skin and handsome physique caught the eyes of many women. But Raphael was not a womanizer. He was devoted to his wife, Joanna, to whom he had been married for fifteen years. They had met in college and the early years of their marriage had been exciting for both of them. But in more recent years, there had developed a growing distance.

Raphael (all names have been changed) had tried to discuss his feelings with Joanna but she didn't want to talk about it until one day when she finally let the words flow, like water rushing down the mountain after a heavy rain. She told Raphael that she was involved with a man at work, that they had been friends for many years and lovers for the past two years.

"I'm sorry," Joanna sobs. "I really am. I didn't want to hurt you. That's why I hadn't told you before. I really don't want to hurt you even now. The other man has moved to New York, and he doesn't want to continue the relationship. I guess I feel heartbroken, but I know I'll get over him someday."

While Joanna feels grief in losing the other man, what she finds most painful is sharing all of this with Raphael. She doesn't want to lose him now. She knows that he has been a devoted husband. At times she feels guilty for what she has done. At other times, she knows that she would do it again given the same circumstances.

Raphael is crushed, but at least now he knows why the distance has been there. Perhaps he would be willing to forgive and work on restoring their relationship if that is what Joanna desires. But one thought plagues him. He remembers that something like this happened earlier in their marriage. Joanna did not get sexually involved with another man, but she did have an emotional attachment with a man she met playing tennis. She told Raphael. The relationship was rather short lived, and Raphael forgave and felt healing had occurred. Now he wonders, *Has this happened more than twice and if I go on with Joanna, will it happen again?*

The disappointment, hurt, anger, and worry are overwhelming at times. He doesn't want a divorce. He loves Joanna in spite of all that's happened, but he cannot live with a repeat performance of what has happened in the past. The pain of living with an unfaithful spouse may at times seem like an incurable infection.

Barbara, on the other hand, is married to an alcoholic husband. He drank some before they got married, but after marriage, drinking became a bigger part of his life. For the past ten years, it has torn their marriage apart. Seeing her husband drunk is disappointment enough, but the verbal abuse that she often receives when he is under the influence of alcohol makes the situation at times unbearable. The pressure is compounded by the fact that his alcoholism has made it difficult for him to hold a job. The pattern has been a new job, new excitement, a commitment to be a success this time. But such hope is always short lived. The drinking returns, the job is lost. Then comes the binge, followed by the drying-out period, and then the job search begins again.

Barbara has a strong religious faith and doesn't believe in divorce. She has talked often about the problem. When her husband is not drinking, he is always apologetic and promises that he can control his drinking next time. But that is also what he promised last time.

"I'm to the point that I don't know what to do now," Barbara told me. "I find my love feelings for him dying and being replaced by pity and anger. I want to respect him. I want to love him. I want to help him, but I don't know how." Thousands can identify with the constant frustration of living with an alcoholic spouse.

I met Daniel in Iowa. He was a pig farmer and extremely successful in his business. "If raising pigs and making money could ensure a good marriage," he said, "I would have one. Dr. Chapman, I consider myself a strong man. I don't usually let things get me down, but my wife's constant criticism has almost destroyed me. Other people can get on my case and I let it roll off like water off a pig's back. But when my wife constantly criticizes me, it's like a dagger in my heart. She's such a negative person not only toward me but toward everyone and toward life in general. She stays depressed a lot of the time. It's almost like she has to bring everybody else down to her level.

"For her, life is miserable and she tries to make my life miserable. I find myself wanting to stay away from the house and not be around her. I know that's not the answer. It has affected our sex life and everything else.

"I don't want to leave my wife. I know she needs help, but I don't know how to help her." Living with a depressed spouse whose only communication is negative and critical can be a constant source of emotional drain and leave one feeling depleted of energy.

Then there is life with a "controller." I knew Jodie in high school, but I had not seen her for many years. She had gone off to college, married, and moved out of state. I was thrilled to see her at one of my marriage seminars. We were catching up on each other when my thrill turned to sadness. She recounted the pain of her twenty-seven-year marriage. Her husband was a hardworking man who had been quite successful in his vocation but quite a failure in providing for Jodie what she had hoped to find in marriage. She had dreamed of a partnership where she and her husband could share thoughts, feelings, desires, and work together as a team in facing life. Her husband, however, came from a family where his father was extremely domineering. Without even realizing it, he had become exactly like his father.

"He controls the money like he is a guard at Fort Knox," Jodie said. "I have to ask for every nickel. Every time I come home, he wants to know where I've been and what I've done. He even checks the odometer on my car and compares it to my account of where I've been. I've given him no reason to think that I'm doing anything behind his back, but he acts like he thinks I'm having an affair or something. He has to have the final decision in everything. Our social life is almost nil because he never wants to do anything with anyone else. He's told our children that he will not pay for their college unless they go to the university of his choice.

"I feel like I'm a bird in a cage. Actually, I feel like a hamster in a cage—I don't have wings anymore. I don't want a divorce, but I don't know how long I can go on living under such pressure." Jodie lives with a controlling husband. She has lost her freedom and is feeling the pain of incarceration.

Then there was Mitzi. She was sitting in my office wearing dark glasses and a long sleeved sweater. It was mid-June. The sun was shining brightly outside. The sunglasses would not have been out of place, but in North Carolina, you don't need a long sleeved sweater in mid-June. She took off her glasses and didn't say a word. I knew I was in the presence of a battered woman. Her eye was black and later I saw that her arms had turned blue from bruises inflicted by her enraged husband.

"Dr. Chapman, I've got to have help," she said. "My husband lost control. He hit me with the telephone repeatedly and he threw a Coke bottle at me. I can't live like this," she said.

"Has anything like this happened before?" I asked. The answer was what I expected.

"Yes, it's happened several times before, but I've never shared it with anyone until now. He always tells me he's sorry and it won't happen again. And I wanted to believe him, but it does happen again. This time is the worst, and I know that I can't take any more chances. I should not have let it go on this long. I need help in deciding what to do." Mitzi was discovering that life with a physical abuser gets progressively worse and, in the end, can be deadly.

A BROKEN WOMAN

It was a beautiful Friday in Birmingham, beautiful that is until I encountered Robbie. She was obviously a broken woman. Tears flowed freely as she said, "I discovered recently that my husband has sexually abused both of our daughters. One is now sixteen and the other is eighteen. Apparently, this has gone on for several years, but I didn't know it until about a month ago. My older daughter finally went for counseling on her college campus. That's what brought it all out. Then she talked to my younger daughter and found out the same thing had been happening with her. As soon as I heard it, I took my younger daughter and went to live with my mother.

"Right now, I hate him and never want to see him again."

"Has he tried to make any contact with you since you left?" I asked.

"Yes, he's called several times but I only talked with him once. He told me that he knew what he did was wrong and he regretted it but that he couldn't take it back now, but he wanted me to know that he was sorry. I don't know, Dr. Chapman. Right now, I'm just so confused." Few things are more disgustingly painful than to discover that your spouse has sexually abused your children.

Then there was Elaine. She was in my office alone, although her husband had come with her for several counseling appointments. This time she said, "He was ashamed to come. He lost his job last week because he got in a fight with a fellow employee."

This had been her husband's pattern for ten years. The longest time he had held a job was eighteen months. He didn't always get in a fight, but he did always get frustrated with the job or the people with whom he worked. His normal pattern was simply to walk off the job with no explanation and simply fade away. The employer typically called Elaine to ask what the problem was and if he were coming back. She would explain that he had told her that he had quit his job; therefore, she assumed that he would not be returning. He would go weeks and sometimes months without work, spending his time sleeping late, watching television, and working out at the local gym.

Elaine had worked a full-time job all ten years of their marriage except for brief times surrounding the births of her two children. When her husband was working, he would help her with the bills, but when he was out of work, she had to carry the whole load. With the tears flowing freely, Elaine said, "Dr. Chapman, I don't know how much longer I can go on." An irresponsible person who is not willing to pull his/her full share of the load puts an undue burden on the spouse. This burden may eventually seem unbearable.

FINDING LOVING SOLUTIONS

Sit in any counselor's office and these are the stories you will hear. Survey the landscape of marriages in this country and you will find it dotted with homes inhabited by people who struggle with similar situations. These are couples who live with real pain. Their problems have no quick fix nor will they go away with time. Hope is often smothered by the magnitude of their problems. These are the kind of problems that I wish to address in this book, including how to deal with a spouse who is unfaithful, alcoholic, controlling, irresponsible, or verbally, physically, or sexually abusive. (In chapter 12 we will look at both the sexually abusive spouse and the spouse who was abused as a child.) For all of these situations, and others, there are loving solutions. Solutions that may preserve the marriage and can make couples feel good about themselves and their spouses.

I am under no illusion that I can give a magic formula to bring healing to all such marriages. However, I do believe, based upon my own experience in counseling, research in the field, and sound moral principles, that there is hope for such marriages.

I believe that in every troubled marriage positive steps can be taken by one or both partners, steps that have the potential for changing the emotional climate between the two of them. In due time they can find answers to their problems. For most of these couples, ultimate solutions will depend not only upon their own actions but upon the support of the religious and therapeutic community in their city. But there is hope—hope for lasting solutions.

This book will explore the nature of these problems and encourage the reader to take steps toward healing rather than sinking deeper into the misery of such relationships. But first, let's look at what has become a rather popular approach to such major marital problems, namely the exit marked *divorce*.

AN HONEST LOOK AT DIVORCE

here are three radical and surely negative approaches to a troubled marriage: suicide, homicide, and divorce. The first two are considered unthinkable by intelligent, mentally healthy people, though sadly enough every year thousands of emotionally disturbed people choose these deadly roads of violence. Most would agree that killing oneself or killing one's spouse are not reasonable or healthy ways of responding to a troubled marriage.

On the other hand, modern man views divorce in a much more positive light. Divorce is seen as a humane way of ending the pain of an unhealthy relationship. While only thousands commit suicide and homicide each year, hundreds of thousands opt for divorce. For the past several years for every two couples who get married, there is one divorce. In the early years of our society, divorce was viewed as sinful and those who experienced it wore its shameful brand for a lifetime. Today, divorce has lost its stigma. We share the details of our divorce as freely as we talk about our vocation. Some have divorced two, three, or more times and are still in search of a happy marriage. Divorce has become the expected procedure if one is not finding fulfillment in a marriage.

Ours has been called the throwaway society. Our foods are packaged in beautiful containers designed to be thrown away. Our cars and household appliances are planned for obsolescence. Our furniture is given to the Goodwill shop not because it is no longer functional but because it is no longer in style. Our unwanted pregnancies are even "thrown away." Business relationships are sustained only so long as they are profitable to the bottom line. Thus, it is no shock that our society has come to accept the concept of a "throwaway marriage." If we are no longer happy with each other and our relationship has run upon hard times, the easy thing is to abandon the relationship and start over.

I wish that I could recommend divorce as an option. When I listen to the deeply pained people whose situations were described in chapter 1, my natural response is to cry, "Get out, get out, get out! Abandon the loser and get on with your life." That would be our approach if we had purchased bad stock. Get out before the stock falls further. But a spouse is not stock. A spouse is a person— a person with emotions, personality, desires, and frustrations; a person to whom we were deeply attracted at one point in our lives; a person for whom we had warm feelings and genuine care. So deeply were we attracted to each other that we made a public commitment of our lives to each other "so long as we both shall live." Now we have a history together. We may even have parented children together.

We cannot walk off from a spouse as easily as we can sell bad stock. Indeed, talk to most adults who have chosen divorce as the answer, and you will find the divorce was preceded by months of intense inner struggle and that the whole ordeal is still viewed as a deeply painful experience.

Yet divorce as a solution to marital problems has proliferated during the final decades of the twentieth century. Divorce now is so widespread that sociologists have been able to complete extensive long-term studies on the effect of divorce upon the couple and their children. Judith S. Wallerstein, director of the largest divorce recovery center in the country, is one of those researchers. She has done extensive research following divorced couples for fifteen years after the divorce with regular interviews and psychiatric measuring inventories, seeking to determine the effects of divorce. Her findings are radically different from what she had supposed. Wallerstein, founder of the Center for the Family in Transition in Corte Madera, California, entered her research with the commonly held idea that divorce is a painful but short-term experience that leads to greater long-term happiness; she theorized that divorce indeed provided a second chance for one who had made a poor marital choice. Her research led her to a far different conclusion.

LASTING SCARS

According to Dr. Wallerstein, the couple and their children never outlive the scars of divorce. Her findings are chronicled in the classic study *Second Chances: Men, Women and Children a Decade After Divorce.*[1]

Couples have various goals, Wallerstein concluded, but they are rarely realized, for divorce greatly complicates things:

> Whatever the reasons behind the decision, most people ending a marriage hope to improve the quality of life for themselves and for their children. They hope to find a new love, a more enriching relationship, a more responsive sexual partner, a more supportive companion, a better provider. Failing that, they hope to establish a single life that will provide greater opportunity for self respect, contentment and serenity, or at the least, less turbulence, intrusiveness, and hurt. People want to believe that divorce will relieve all their stresses—back we go to square one and begin our lives anew. But divorce does not wipe the slate clean. . . . Few adults anticipate accurately what lies ahead when they decide to divorce. Life is almost always more arduous and more complicated than they expect.[2]

Here are some of the revealing statistics of Wallerstein's fifteen-year study, and the researcher's response to the findings:

Incredibly, one-half of the women and one-third of the men are still intensely angry at their former spouses, despite the passage of years. . . . To our astonishment, divorce continues to occupy a central, emotional position in the lives of many adults, ten and fifteen years later. . . . A third of the women and a quarter of the men feel that life is unfair, disappointing and lonely. I knew that divorce is not an event that can be gotten over if one simply waits long enough, but even I was surprised at the staying power of feelings after divorce. . . . There is no evidence that time automatically diminishes feelings or memories; that hurt and depression are overcome; or that jealousy, anger, and outrage will vanish. . . . People go on living, but just because they have lived ten more years does not mean they have recovered from the hurt.[3]

And what of the children of divorce? When parents divorce, children lose something that is fundamental to their development—the family structure. Typically, children feel intensely rejected when their parents divorce. Wallerstein agreed, noting, "Children get angry at their parents for violating the unwritten rules of parenthood—parents are supposed to make sacrifices for children, not the other way around. Some keep their anger hidden for years out of fear of upsetting parents or for fear of retribution and punishment; others show it." She concludes: "Children do not perceive divorce as a second chance, and this is part of their suffering. They feel that their childhood has been lost forever. . . . Although children need parents and parents want to continue good relationships with their children, parent-child relationships are forever altered by divorce."[4]

Because we are creatures of memory and relationships, we carry the pain of broken relationships for a lifetime. Children whose parents have divorced put themselves in a different category, referring to themselves as "children of divorce." They recognize that the parents' divorce has made its mark on them emotionally. Many fear for their own future marital happiness and, in fact, the divorce rate for children of divorce is higher than those whose parents remain together. Only a small percentage of divorced individuals claim to have found greater happiness in a second or third marriage. In fact, whereas the divorce rate in first marriages is 40 percent, the divorce rate in second marriages is 60 percent and in third marriages, 75 percent. Thus, the prospects of finding a healthier marriage diminish with each remarriage. The hope of the grass being greener on the other side is just a myth.

Divorce, unlike death, does not end the partners' contact with each other. Most end up living in the same city, particularly if children are involved. Each parent wants to continue a relationship with the children; thus, they find themselves having regular contact with each other whether they want it or not. The nature of these contacts often keep the wounds of a broken relationship oozing with infection for years. Financially caring for the children is an obligation that cannot be discarded by a caring parent. Differences of opinion on handling the financial needs of the children often becomes a constant source of irritation between ex-spouses. Then there are the piano recitals, the ball games, the graduations, and the weddings—all of which are filled with tension as two parents seek to be there for their children while not being there for each other. Many of life's joyous occasions are dampened by the attitudes of two ex-spouses who have different opinions about how the celebration should be conducted.

Nor is divorce a pretty picture financially. The Wallerstein study found that 73 percent of divorced women experience a decline in standard of living after divorce.[5] Evelyn was sitting in my office two years after her divorce from Bill. "Our marriage was bad," she said, "but our divorce is even worse. I still have all the responsibilities I had when we were married and now, I have less time and less money. When we were married, I worked part time to help out with the bills. Now I have to work full time, which gives me less time with the girls. When I am at home, I seem to be more irritable. I find myself snapping at the girls when they don't respond immediately to my request.

"I hate being the kind of mother I am, and I get no support from Bill. When he does take the girls, which is about every third weekend, he makes it a party time for them—no chores, no work, no responsibilities; just fun with Dad. They come home resenting me for expecting them to do anything. Sometimes I wish that he would just get out of our lives, but I know that the girls need to have a relationship with their father. It doesn't seem to get any easier, and I don't see any light at the end of the tunnel." Thousands of divorced moms can identify with Evelyn. Divorce doesn't treat them fairly. The stresses of meeting the physical and emotional needs of their children at times seem overwhelming.

Not all who undergo divorce experience such hardship; yet, all find the adjustments painful, even when divorce is followed by remarriage. Wayne was all smiles when he said to me, "I finally met the love of my life. We are going to get married in June. I've never been happier. She has two children, and I adore them. When I was going through my divorce, I never dreamed that I would be happy again. I believe now that I'm about to get my life back on track." Wayne had been divorced three years at the time of our conversation. However, six months after his marriage to Beverly, he was back in my office complaining about his inability to get along with Beverly and her children.

"It's like I'm an outsider," he said. "She always puts the children before me. And when I seek to discipline the children, she takes their side and disagrees with me. I can't spend a dime without her approval. I've never been so miserable in my life. How did I let myself get into this mess?" Wayne is experiencing the common struggles of establishing a "blended family."

LIFE AFTER DIVORCE

There are no "and they all lived happily ever after" divorces. The effects of divorce linger for a lifetime. This is not to say that there is no life after divorce. It is to say that life after divorce is always impacted by life before the divorce. Because the marriage relationship is unique among human relationships and involves deep emotional ties on the part of the husband and wife (at least at some juncture in the relationship, because they have shared their lives with each other for a period of time), there is no "walking away without pain." The good and bad memories of the past will be ours forever, and whatever contact we may have with each other in the future, the reality of our problems will still exist.

Through the years I have counseled enough divorced persons to know that while divorce removes some pressures, it creates a host of others. I am not naive enough to suggest that divorce can be eliminated from the human landscape. I am saying that divorce should be the last possible alternative. It should be preceded by every effort at reconciling differences, dealing with issues, and solving problems. Far too many couples in our society have opted for divorce too soon and at too great a price. I believe that many divorced couples could have reconciled if they had sought and found proper help. Thus, the focus of this book is not on suicide, homicide, or divorce but on something I believe offers far more hope. It's what I call "reality living."

Reality living focuses on positive action that one individual can take to stimulate constructive change in a relationship. In the next chapter I will give you the basic principles of this approach and in the following chapters, we will apply these principles to various kinds of troubled marriages.

NOTES

1. Wallerstein's report, based on a trailblazing longitudinal study of the effects of divorce, was published in 1989. See Judith Wallerstein and Sandra Blakeslee, *Second Chances* (New York: Ticknor and Fields, 1989).
2. Wallerstein, *Second Chances*, 3–4.
3. Ibid., 29–30.
4. Ibid., 11–19.
5. Ibid., 19.

CHAPTER THREE

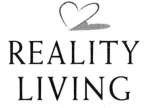

REALITY
LIVING

*L*ook at the following four statements. Which of them are true?

1. My state of mind is determined by my environment.
2. People cannot change.
3. When you are in a bad marriage, there are only two options —resign yourself to a life of misery or get out.
4. Some situations are hopeless.

If you answered "true" to any of these, please read on. In fact, all four statements are false; they are commonly held myths.

Unfortunately, many people in troubled marriages base their lives upon commonly held myths. If you or someone you love has a troubled marriage, it's time to practice reality living. Reality living identifies myths that have held us captive and exposes them for what they are. We can break their bands as we begin to base our actions upon truth rather than myth. In fact, *reality living* means taking responsibility for my own thoughts, feelings, and actions. It requires an honest appraisal of my life situation and refuses to shift the blame for my unhappiness to others.

EXPOSING FOUR MYTHS

However, those who accept any of the four myths above will act accordingly, so that their actions become a part of the problem rather than a part of the solution. Let's look at the outcome of accepting and acting upon each of these myths.

Myth Number One: My state of mind is determined by my environment. The commonly held view of our day is that we are victims of our environment. This view is expressed in the following statements. If I grew up in a loving supportive family, I will be a loving supportive person. If I grew up in a dysfunctional family, then I am destined to failure in relationships. If I am married to an alcoholic husband, I will live a miserable life. My mental emotional state is determined by the actions of my spouse.

This kind of approach to life renders one helpless in a hostile environment. It is accompanied by feelings of hopelessness and often leads to depression. In a troubled marriage, this victim mentality leads the spouse to conclude, *My life is miserable and my only hope is the death of my spouse or divorce.* Many people daydream of both. Our environment certainly affects who we are, but it does not control us. Rather than being helpless victims, we can overcome an environment cluttered with obstacles, whether blindness or polio—consider Helen Keller and Franklin Roosevelt—or an alcoholic parent, whose abuse has influenced your attitudes in marriage. The environment may influence, but it need not dictate—nor destroy—your marriage and your life.

Myth Number Two: People cannot change. This myth purports that once people reach adulthood, personality traits and behavior patterns are set in concrete. Those who believe this myth reason that if their spouse was sexually active with multiple partners before marriage and has been sexually unfaithful after marriage, that they are addicted to this behavior and cannot change. If a spouse has been irresponsible in money management for the first fifteen years of marriage, it is reasoned that he or she will always be financially irresponsible. If your spouse has verbally abused you for ten years, you conclude he or she will be a verbal abuser for life.

Accepting this myth as truth often leads to feelings of futility and hopelessness. This myth fails to reckon with the reality of human freedom. The fact is libraries are filled with accounts of people who have made radical changes in their behavior patterns. From St. Augustine, who once lived for pleasure and thought his desires were inescapable, to Charles Colson, the Watergate criminal who repented and began an international agency to offer prisoners spiritual help, volumes of biographies testify against the validity of this myth. People can and do change, and often the changes are dramatic.

Myth Number Three: When you are in a bad marriage, there are only two options— resign yourself to a life of misery or get out. This myth limits one's horizons to two equally devastating alternatives. Once the choice is made between these alternatives, the individual becomes a prisoner of his choice. Thousands of people live in these self-made prisons because they believed the myth of limited choices.

Shannon and David had believed this myth. For fifteen years they had experienced misery and contemplated divorce, but as they left my office after six months of counseling, David said, "I used to leave your office with rage in my heart toward her. Today I leave realizing what a wonderful wife I have." A smile spread across Shannon's face as she spoke. "Dr. Chapman, I never dreamed that I could love him again and we could have the marriage we have." Obviously, Shannon and David had broken the bondage of this myth.

Myth Number Four: Some situations are hopeless. This myth is normally coupled with the corollary myth " . . . And my situation is one of these." The person who accepts this myth reasons: *Perhaps there is hope for others, but my marriage is hopeless. It has gone on too long; the hurt is too deep; the damage is irreversible. There is no hope.* This kind of thinking leads to depression and sometimes suicide.

I listened with tears as Lisa, a thirty-five-year-old mother, shared her story of watching her father murder her mother and then turn the gun on himself. Lisa was ten when she experienced this tragedy. Fortunately, she had worked through the trauma of that childhood experience, but she still acutely realized the senselessness of that hopeless act. I personally wonder how many of the homicides and suicides in this nation arise out of the hearts of those who have believed the myth that their situation was hopeless.

EMBRACING SIX REALITIES

Reality living refuses to believe these myths and chooses rather to face life with a far more positive spirit. What are the postulates of reality living as they apply to troubled marriages? Let me share six truths that can give direction to any troubled marriage.

Reality Number One: I am responsible for my own attitude. Reality living approaches life with the assumption that I am responsible for my own state of mind. Trouble is inevitable, but misery is optional. Attitude has to do with the way I choose to think about things. It has to do with one's focus. Two men looked through prison bars—one saw the mud, the other saw the stars. Two people were in a troubled marriage—one cursed, the other prayed. The difference always is attitude.

Negative thinking tends to beget negative thinking. Focus on how terrible the situation is, and it will get worse. Focus on one positive thing, and another will appear. In the darkest night of a troubled marriage, there is always a flickering light. Focus on that light and it will eventually flood the room. Socrates knew the importance of attitude when he advised the men of his day, "By all means marry; if you get a good wife, you will become happy; if you get a bad one, you will become a philosopher."[1] I have met numerous men and women who have become good philosophers. They have learned to think positively in the midst of troubled marriages.

Wendy said, "My husband hasn't had a full-time job in three years. The good part is not being able to afford cable TV. We've done a lot more talking on Monday nights." She went on to say, "These three years have been tough but we have learned a lot. Our philosophy has been 'Let's see how many things we can do without that everybody else thinks they have to have.' It's amazing how many things you can do without. It's been a challenge, but we are going to make the most of it."

Three weeks after I met Wendy, I encountered Lou Ann. She was at the point of mental and physical exhaustion. Her husband had been out of work for ten months and was working a part-time job while looking for full-time employment. However, Lou Ann had been biting her nails for ten months. She was certain that they would lose everything they owned; she decried the fact that they could not afford cable television and talked about how difficult it was to operate with only one car. Every day she lived on the cutting edge of despair.

The difference between Wendy and Lou Ann was basically a matter of attitude. Their problems were very similar, but their attitudes were very different, and that difference had a profound impact upon their physical and emotional well-being.

The challenge to a positive mental attitude is not a contemporary idea. It is found clearly in the first-century writings of Saul of Tarsus: "Do not be anxious about anything, but in everything, by prayer and petition, with thanksgiving, present your requests to God. And the peace of God, which transcends all understanding, will guard your hearts and minds. . . . Finally, brothers, whatever is true, whatever is noble, whatever is right, whatever is pure, whatever is lovely, whatever is admirable—if anything is excellent or praiseworthy—think about such things."[2] This first postulate of reality living is that I am responsible for my own attitude. The second is closely associated with the first.

Reality Number Two: Attitude affects actions. The reason attitudes are so important is that they affect my actions: behavior and words. If I have a pessimistic, defeatist, negative attitude it will be expressed in negative words and behavior. At that point, I become a part of the problem rather than a part of the solution. The reality is that I may not be able to control my environment: sickness, alcoholic spouse, teenager on drugs, mother who abandoned me, father who abused me, spouse who is irresponsible, aging parents, etc.; but I am responsible for what I do within my environment. My attitude will greatly influence my behavior.

Clearly Wendy and Lou Ann demonstrated this reality. With her positive attitude, Wendy had done several things over the past three years to enhance the climate of her marriage. She had given her husband affirming words when he got discouraged in his job search. She had assured him that the right job would come and in the meantime, they would make it on his part-time job and her part-time job. She had suggested that they collect aluminum cans to obtain "fun" money. At first her husband had resisted the idea, thinking it humiliating. Eventually, though, he liked the idea, and they enthusiastically collected cans not only on the highways when they took their evening walk, but also through several local establishments with whom they arranged to pick up their cans. Within three months, they had built up their volume so that every week, they could go out to eat and attend a movie or some other recreational activity. Neither of them felt guilty about spending this money to have fun because they had created it for that purpose. Wendy's attitude had led her to positive creative actions.

On the other hand, Lou Ann had been verbally critical of her husband for ten months. When he came home without a job, she asked him, "What did you do wrong this time?" She had told all her friends how disappointed she was in her husband. He often overheard her on the telephone saying such things as, "I don't know what we're going to do if he doesn't get a job soon." Her husband had a part-time job, but she did not. Her reasoning was "We can't make a living on part-time jobs, so why bother?" She spent most of her time sleeping, watching television, and visiting with her friends. Her marriage was in serious trouble. Her negative attitudes led to negative actions that compounded the problem. Attitude affects actions, and actions influence others. Which brings us to the third reality.

Reality Number Three: I cannot change others, but I can influence others. The two parts of this reality must never be separated. That I cannot change my spouse is an often recited truth, but that I can and do influence my spouse is a truth often overlooked. Because we are individuals and because we are free, no one can force us to change our thoughts or behavior. On the other hand, because people are relational creatures, they are influenced by all to whom they relate. Advertisers make millions of dollars each year because of this reality. They do not make us buy their product, but they do influence us. Otherwise, they would drop their advertisements.

This reality has profound implications for marriage. I must acknowledge that I cannot change my spouse. I cannot make her stop certain behaviors or start certain behaviors. (Though she may change herself [see myth two]). I can neither control the words that come from her mouth, nor can I control the way she thinks or feels. I can make requests of my spouse, but I cannot be assured that she will respond positively to my requests.

When we fail to understand this reality, we are likely to fall into the trap of seeking to manipulate our spouse. The idea behind manipulation is that if I will do this, my spouse will be forced to do that. Manipulation may involve positive stimuli as well as negative stimuli. If I can make her (or him) happy enough, she will respond to my request. Or if I can make her miserable enough, she will respond to my request. All efforts at manipulation will ultimately fail for one simple reason. We are free. The moment we realize the individual—including our spouse—is controlling us by manipulation, we will rebel. None of us wants to be controlled by our spouses.

However, our inability to change our spouses must be laid alongside our ability to influence them—for better or for worse. All married couples influence each other every day. This is done by our attitudes and actions. This influence is exerted every time we encounter each other throughout the day. Your spouse walks in the room in the afternoon, gives you a hug and kiss, and says, "I love you. I've missed you today." With those simple actions and words, he has influenced you in a positive way. On the other hand, if your spouse walks into the house, goes straight to his computer room or walks out on the patio to drink a Coke, and fails to acknowledge your presence, or if he walks in and gives you critical words about your appearance or behavior, he has influenced you in a negative way. Chances are your response to those two encounters will be vastly different. One tends to influence you to respond positively; the other influences you to respond negatively.

This reality of our influence upon each other happens every day. Every action and every word influences our spouse—for better or for worse. This reality has a downside in that the words and behavior of your spouse may cause you tremendous pain, hurt, discouragement, etc. But this reality is also a profound asset; it gives you the power of influencing your spouse toward positive change.

Over the years, I have tested this reality with numerous individuals in troubled marriages. When an individual is willing to choose a positive attitude that leads to positive actions, the change in his or her spouse has often been radical. One lady said, "I can't believe what has happened to my husband. I never dreamed that he could be as loving and kind as he has been for the last two months. This is more change than I ever anticipated." The reality of the power of positive influence holds tremendous potential for troubled marriages.

Reality Number Four: My actions are not controlled by my emotions. In the last three decades with the rise of popular psychology, especially through the mass media, Western society has given an undue emphasis to human emotions. In fact, emotions have become our guiding star. Our songs and movies are filled with such themes as "If it feels good, do it"; "I must be true to my emotions"; "When I'm with you, I feel so good"; "I just don't love her anymore." The search for self-understanding has led us to the conclusion that "you *are* what you *feel*" and that authentic living is being "true to your feelings."

When applied to a troubled marriage, this philosophy advises, "If you don't have love feelings for your spouse any longer, admit it and get out of the marriage. If you feel hurt and angry, you would be hypocritical to say or do something kind to your spouse." This philosophy fails to reckon with the reality that man is more than his emotions.

The truth is we experience life through the five senses: sight, sound, smell, taste, and touch. All that we experience comes through one of the five senses. In response to what we experience through the senses, we have *thoughts, feelings, desires,* and *actions.* Notice that only one of these four responses to our senses—feelings—bears directly on our emotions, so we need not have emotions control us.

In our *thoughts,* we interpret what we experience through the five senses. We see dirty dishes in the sink at 10:30 P.M. and we interpret that our spouse is lazy. We hear our spouse on the telephone say to someone, "I love you too," and we interpret that she is having an affair. We see and hear our spouse mowing the grass, and we interpret that he is a responsible individual.

Accompanying our thoughts will be *emotions.* Believing that our spouse is lazy, we may feel disappointment, anger, and frustration. Believing that our spouse is having an affair may stimulate hurt, anger, and bitterness. Believing our spouse to be a responsible person, we feel grateful, encouraged, and happy.

In response to these thoughts and feelings, we have *desires*. The dirty dishes may create a desire to give our spouse a lecture on irresponsibility. The thought of an affair may give us the desire to cry in despair, lash out in anger, or walk out the door and never return. Seeing our spouse mowing the grass may give us the desire to take him a glass of lemonade or to express verbal appreciation when he has completed the job.

Eventually, we take *action*. Based on our thoughts, emotions, and desires, we do something. If we allow our negative emotions and desires to control our actions, we will typically make the situation worse because our action will be negative, which in turn will stimulate a negative response in our spouse. If, on the other hand, we take a reasoned approach and ask ourselves, "What is the best thing to do in this situation?" we are far more likely to take positive action.

Facing the dirty dishes at 10:30 P.M., I may decide to wash them and tell my spouse, "I love you so much I didn't want you to face those dirty dishes in the morning." To the telephone conversation that ended with the words "I love you too," I might choose to say to my spouse, "I assume you were talking to your mother?" to which my spouse may respond, "No, I was talking to Julie. She is spending the night with Mindy."

When your spouse finishes mowing the yard, you may give him/her a glass of lemonade and say, "You are such a wonderful person. I don't know what I'd do without you." On the other hand, you may choose to say, "It's about time you mowed the grass. It was beginning to look like a jungle." One need not be a psychologist to understand that our actions either enhance or destroy relationships.

The reality is that our actions are far more important than our emotions and, in fact, our actions will affect our emotions. I may feel depressed. Life seems heavy. A friend calls and asks if I'd like to join him for a Coke float at Mayberry's. My emotions are negative; my desire is to lie on the couch and forget the world, but I choose to say yes. Two hours later, my emotions have changed and the world looks much brighter.

My behavior influenced my emotions. This is true on the personal level and it is also true in relationships. My actions influence your emotions. If I give you a kind word or perform a loving act, chances are your emotions will be positive. In relationships, actions are far more important than emotions, and actions need not be controlled by emotions. If I allow my negative emotions to control my behavior, I will feel even more negative. But if I choose to take positive actions in spite of my negative emotions, my emotions are likely to change, and my actions may have a positive influence on you.

Viktor Frankl discovered the power of positive actions in the midst of German concentration camps. "We who lived in the concentration camps can remember the men who walked through the huts comforting others, giving away their last piece of bread. They may have been few in number, but they offer sufficient proof that everything can be taken from a man but one thing: the last of his freedoms—to choose one's attitude in any given set of circumstances, to choose one's own way."[3] The men who chose to do such loving acts were not motivated by emotions but rather by their attitudes. Their actions affected the emotions and attitudes of fellow prisoners. Emotions are extremely flimsy and can change momentarily. They are not a firm foundation on which to build life.

Those who object that it is hypocritical to take positive action when one has negative feelings are operating on the assumption that the true self is determined by our emotions. I am suggesting that is a false premise and to the degree that it has permeated Western thinking, it has been detrimental to family relationships. In other areas of life, we often go against our emotions. For example, if I would get out of bed only on the mornings that I "feel" like getting out of bed, I'd have bed sores. The fact is, almost every morning I go against my feelings, get up, do something, and later feel good about having gotten out of bed. The same principle is true in relationships.

In our efforts to be true to our emotions, we have taken destructive actions that have compounded our emotional sense of well-being. The more positive road is to acknowledge our negative emotions but not to follow them. We do not deny that we feel disappointed, frustrated, angry, hurt, apathetic, or bitter, but we refuse to let these emotions control our actions. We choose the higher road by asking such questions as "What is best? What is right? What is good? What is loving?" We allow our actions to be controlled by these noble thoughts. Taking such positive actions hold the potential for bringing healing to a relationship and restoring positive feelings to both partners.

I am not suggesting that emotions are unimportant. They are indicators that things are going well or not so well in our relationship. Positive emotions encourage me to positive actions. Negative emotions conversely encourage me toward negative actions. But if I understand that negative actions will make things worse and positive actions hold the potential for making things better, I will always choose the high road. I am always influenced by my emotions, but I need not be controlled by them.

This reality has profound implications for a troubled marriage. It means that I can do and say positive things to my spouse in spite of the fact that I have strong negative emotions. To take such positive action does not deny that our marriage is in serious trouble. It does not overlook the problems, but it chooses to take steps that hold potential for positive change rather than allowing negative behavior to escalate.

The good news is that we don't have to have loving, warm feelings to take loving actions. One husband said, "She has disappointed me so much and hurt me so deeply that I have no desire to do anything good for her." He is stating clearly his emotional state and his lack of desire for positive action. He was not being hypocritical when he added, "But understanding the power of positive actions, I will choose to wash and vacuum her car because I know that is something she would like for me to do." One positive action does not heal the hurt of a lifetime, but it is a step in the right direction. A series of positive actions holds the potential for turning the tide in a troubled marriage.

Reality Number Five: Admitting my imperfections does not mean that I am a failure. Most troubled marriages include a stone wall between husband and wife, built over many years. Each stone represents an event in the past where one of them has failed the other. These are the things about which people talk when they sit in the counseling office. The husband complains, "She has been critical of my performance on the job or as a father. . . . She has failed to give me any words of appreciation and affirmation for my hard work. She has put me down in front of the children." On the other hand, she gripes that "He is married to his job and has no time for me. . . . He often ignores me when he comes home, and he expects me to be a slave around the house while he watches football on television."

On and on the list goes. Each recounts what the other has done to make the marriage miserable. This wall stands as a monument to self-centered living, and it's a barrier to marital intimacy.

Demolishing this emotional wall is essential for rebuilding a troubled marriage. Destroying the wall requires both individuals to admit that they are imperfect and have failed each other. I am not implying that the responsibility for the wall is equally distributed between the husband and the wife. Many times, one is more at fault than the other; but the fact is that neither has been perfect.

To acknowledge your imperfections does not mean you're a failure; it is rather to admit that you're human. As humans, you and I have the potential for loving, kind, and good behavior, but we also have the potential for self-centered, destructive behavior. For all of us, our marital history is a mixed bag of good and bad behavior. Admitting our past failures and asking for forgiveness is one of the most liberating of all human experiences. The fact is your spouse knows that you have failed, and you know that you have failed.

When I admit my failure and request forgiveness, I am tearing the wall down on my side. My spouse may readily forgive me or may be reluctant to do so, but I have done the most positive thing I can do about past failures. I cannot remove them nor can I remove all of their results, but I can acknowledge them and request forgiveness.

Many people have found the following statements to be helpful in verbalizing their confession of past failures:

"I've been thinking about us and I realize that in the past, I have not been the perfect husband/wife. In many ways I have failed you and hurt you. I am sincerely sorry for these failures. I hope that you will be able to forgive me for these. I sincerely want to be a better husband/wife. And with God's help, I want to make the future different."

Whether your spouse verbalizes forgiveness or has some less enthusiastic response, you have taken the first step in tearing the wall down between the two of you. If the hurt has been deep, your spouse may question your sincerity. He or she may even say, "I've heard that line before," or "I'm not sure that I can forgive you." Whatever the response, you have planted in his or her mind the idea that the future is going to be different. If, in fact, you begin to make positive changes as a spouse, the day may come when your partner will freely forgive past failures. Until then, you concentrate on making positive changes.

To admit your own past failures does not mean that you are accepting all the responsibility for your troubled marriage. It does mean that you are no longer using your spouse's failures as an excuse for your own. You are stepping up to take full responsibility for your own failures and you are doing the most responsible thing you can do by acknowledging them and asking forgiveness. In so doing, you are paving the road of hope for a new future.

I am fully aware that most of the people who read this book will read it alone. In a troubled marriage, it is unrealistic to think that husband and wife will sit down together and work through a book. That may happen in a healthy marriage but not in a deeply troubled marriage. Therefore, if you are reading this book, I want to encourage you to tear down the wall on your side. You may feel that the bulk of the wall is on your spouse's side and that may be true. But the reality is that you cannot tear down his or her wall; you can tear down only the wall on your side. However small it may be, it is a step in the right direction and it opens the potential for positive actions on your part. It lets your spouse know that you are consciously thinking about your marriage relationship.

The sixth reality that helps our marriages is probably the most important. It's so important that I want to highlight it in a chapter of its own. Let's turn now to chapter 5 and the final reality: the power of love to help us in our marriages.

NOTES

1. As quoted in Billy and Janice Hughey, *A Rainbow of Hope* (El Reno, Okla.: Rainbow Studios, 1994), 190.
2. Philippians 4:6–8, New International Version.
3. As quoted in George Sweeting, *Who Said That?* (Chicago: Moody, 1995), 57.

THE POWER
OF LOVE

*J*ust released after nineteen hard years in a cold, dank prison, Jean Valjean finds every innkeeper refusing him lodging because of his past. Though he has money and is polite enough, no one permits him to stop; the word is out: he is an ex-convict. After a local resident rejects Valjean's request for merely a bowl of soup and shelter in a garden shed, the weary traveler faces a chilling wind and decides to improvise. He ducks into a small hut in another garden and finds a bed of straw awaiting. No sooner does he begin to loosen his knapsack than he hears growling just outside. There, at the opening, is the head of an enormous bulldog—he had entered a doghouse!

Valjean leaves quickly, but not before the angry dog adds another rip to the man's tattered clothes. Valjean escapes the garden, clears its fence, and eventually sits upon a large stone. "I am not even a dog!" he says.

The humiliated traveler resumes his wandering. He soon locates a stone bench in front of a printing office and accepts it for his bed. He has just lain down when a kindly woman appears, telling him free lodging exists across the square at a little low house. Valjean goes knocking, and he finds a warm welcome in the home of Bishop Myriel. The kindly priest gives the bitter ex-convict food, clothing, a free night's lodging, and helps Valjean regain his strength. The traveler is stunned by the host's hospitality and care.

After a short, deep sleep, the ex-convict awakes. He sneaks into the kitchen, steals the silver from his benefactor, and flees into the night. The French authorities arrest Valjean with the silver and return him to the priest, ready to jail the criminal once more. Valjean is stunned when Bishop Myriel intercedes. "And you brought him back here?" Myriel tells the police, "It is all a mistake."

Then the bishop tells the convict, "My friend, before you go away, here are your candlesticks; take them." Myriel pulls the two silver candlesticks from the mantle and gives them to the ex-convict.

The act of love and forgiveness changes Valjean. He becomes an industrious worker, and later runs a factory where he is known for his compassion and fairness to the workers. Townspeople ask him to run for mayor and he wins the election. His charity to all is well known.

Les Misérables, the story of how convict Jean Valjean received the unconditional love of a priest and opened himself to love others, moved readers in the nineteenth century and moves theatergoers today as a popular stage musical. Such giving and sacrificial love makes for a powerful story, and indeed *Les Misérables* is considered a classic novel by Victor Hugo. But the love displayed by the bishop and later by Jean Valjean is not just a fairy tale.

Such love *can* exist. And it shows the final principle of reality living in action. It is probably the most important reality to help a troubled marriage. For when we give love, those who need it most—those closest to us in our families—are restored and have a fresh hope.

Here is reality number six: *Love is the most powerful weapon for good in the world.* The French novelist Hugo described how the unconditional love of a priest opened convict Jean Valjean to return love, and even to love others sacrificially: Valjean would do good even when it meant loss of personal comfort, and seemed to threaten his own best interests. Hugo once wrote, "The supreme happiness of life is the conviction that we are loved."[1]

Many agree with the novelist. Sigmund Freud said, "Love is the first requirement of mental health."[2] William James said, "The deepest principle in human nature is the craving to be appreciated."[3] Religious and secular leaders today agree that love holds a central place in man's search for meaning. It is unfortunate that in the modern world the focus has been more on receiving love than giving love.

Most of the couples who sit in my office talk about the lack of love, affection, and appreciation they have received from their spouse through the years. Their emotional love tanks are empty and they are pleading for love. I am deeply sympathetic with this need. I believe love is man's deepest emotional need. The difficulty in a troubled marriage is that we are focusing on receiving love rather than giving love. Many husbands say, "If she would just be a little more affectionate then I could be responsive to her; but when she gives me no affection, I just want to stay away from her." He is waiting for love before he loves. However, someone must take the initiative. Why must it be the other person?

The final principle for reality living declares love to be the most powerful weapon for good, and that especially applies in marriage. The problem for many husbands and wives is that we have thought of love as an emotion. In reality, love is an attitude with appropriate behavior. It affects the emotions, but it is not in itself an emotion. Love is the attitude that says "I choose to look out for your interests. How may I help you?" Then love is expressed in behavior.

LOVE AS ACTION

The so-called Golden Rule reads: "Do to others what you would have them do to you."[4] This is in fact a definition of love. Love is action that grows out of thoughts. Love is the action which grows out of the attitude "I'm going to do something good for him/her." Love is doing for the other person what you wish he or she would do for you.

The fact that love is action rather than emotion means that I can love my spouse even when I do not have warm emotional feelings for him/her. You and I may have negative emotions and still choose to love our spouses. That is why in the first century Paul, the apostle, wrote to husbands "Love your wives, just as Christ loved the church and gave himself up for her [by willingly dying on a cross]."[5] In another of his letters, Paul challenged the older women to "train the younger women to love their husbands."[6] Love can be learned because it is not an emotion.

When we understand that love is basically a way of thinking and behaving, we can then love our spouse, even when we have negative emotions toward him or her. Our loving actions tend to stimulate positive emotions in our spouse. These emotions encourage our mate to reciprocate. When our spouses express loving actions to us, our emotions respond and we begin to feel warmly toward them. Thus the emotion of love grows out of loving actions.

Emotional warmth can be reborn in a marriage, but it is the result of loving actions. If we simply wait for warm emotions to return, we may wait in vain; but if we choose loving actions toward our spouse, we are setting in motion the cycle which stimulates warm emotions.

SPEAKING YOUR SPOUSE'S LOVE LANGUAGE

Part of the problem in demonstrating our love is that we have failed to understand that husbands and wives speak different "love languages." After twenty-five years of counseling, I am convinced there are only five basic languages of love. These are ways we can communicate love to our spouses. They are:

1. *Words of affirmation*—verbally affirming them for the good things they do.
2. *Quality time*—giving them your undivided attention. This may involve going out to eat or taking a walk together or an extended weekend with just the two of you.
3. *Receiving gifts*—a gift says "He/She was thinking about me."
4. *Acts of service*—doing things for your spouse, anything that you know is meaningful to him/her.
5. *Physical touch*—kissing, embracing, a pat on the back, holding hands, sexual intercourse.

All of these communicate love. Out of these five, one is *your* primary love language. One of these five speaks more deeply to you on the emotional level than the others. When love is expressed to you in that way, you understand that you are loved. Seldom, however, do the husband and wife have the same love language. By nature, we tend to speak our own language. If quality time makes me feel loved, then that's what I try to give my spouse. But if that is not his/her primary language, it will not mean to my mate what it would mean to me.

For example, if your husband's love language is words of affirmation and you are giving him gifts as an expression of love, he may reason, "Why do you keep spending our money this way? We can't afford these gifts." You feel rebuffed and wonder why he is so cold to your expressions of love. If, on the other hand, your spouse's language is receiving gifts and you give words of affirmation, your spouse may well say, "Cut the words, please. Where are the gifts? Talk is cheap. You never give me anything." Both may be sincere, but they are expressing love in their own language, not the language of their spouse.[7] So you need to know, and then speak, your spouse's primary love language.

This simple concept, which I have shared in marriage seminars and the book *The Five Love Languages*, has helped thousands of couples learn to communicate love in a way that best stimulates warm emotions inside the spouse. Discovering your spouse's primary love language and choosing to speak it on a regular basis has tremendous potential for changing the emotional climate in a marriage.

Love is the most powerful weapon for good not only in the world but in a troubled marriage. When we choose to reach out with a loving attitude and loving actions toward our spouse in spite of past failures, we are creating a climate where conflicts can be resolved, wrongs can be confessed, and a marriage can be reborn. Reality living says, "I will choose the road of love because its potential is far greater than the road of hate." Martin Luther King Jr. said, "I have decided to stick with love. Hate is too great a burden to bear."[8] If we do not choose to love people more than they deserve, then none of us will ever express love.

LOVING SOLUTIONS

SIX REALITIES FOR TROUBLED MARRIAGES

This powerful weapon called love is the final aspect of reality living. All six elements point the way to loving solutions in our marriages that can bring husbands and wives back together. Again, the six realities are:

1. I am responsible for my own attitude.
2. Attitude affects actions.
3. I cannot change others, but I can influence others.
4. My actions are not controlled by my emotions.
5. Admitting my imperfections does not mean that I am a failure.
6. Love is the most powerful weapon for good in the world.

These six realities hold tremendous potential for troubled marriages. In the chapters that follow, we will look at examples of deeply troubled marriages that have applied these realities and found healing. I am deeply sympathetic with those who feel that there is no hope for their marriage. I fully understand how we can come to the end of our rope emotionally. Our energies are drained from past efforts, none of which have been successful. But let's not assume that past failures must be repeated in the future. With a new set of guidelines and a willingness to take action, there is hope for troubled marriages. I am convinced that there is always some positive step that can be taken even in the most troubled marriage. It is by means of positive steps that a marriage is changed. Even "baby steps" will get us to our goal if we take enough of them.

The approach in the chapters that follow is to help you discover positive steps you can take to make a difference in your marriage. I understand that you wish your spouse would join you in working on the marriage; that is probably an unrealistic hope at the moment, but that does not mean that the marriage is hopeless. One person can make a tremendous impact on a marriage relationship if he or she has the right guidance and takes the right steps. One person must always take the initiative. Perhaps that person will be you. You will never know the power of reality living until you try it.

NOTES

1. As quoted by Billy Graham in George Sweeting, *Who Said That?* (Chicago: Moody, 1995), 313.
2. Ibid.
3. As quoted in Sweeting, *Who Said That?*, 171.
4. Matthew 7:12, New International Version (NIV).
5. Ephesians 5:25, NIV. According to the biblical writers, Jesus Christ's death by crucifixion was done willingly to pay for the sins of men and women. It was an act of sacrificial love to bring estranged men and women back to God. See Matthew 16:21; John 10:17–18; Romans 5:6–10.
6. Titus 2:4, NIV.
7. For a fuller explanation of this concept, see Gary Chapman, *The Five Love Languages: How to Express Heartfelt Commitment to Your Spouse* (Chicago: Northfield, 1995).
8. As quoted in Sweeting, *Who Said That?*, 306.

UNDERSTANDING THE HIDDEN SELF

*J*eff and his wife, Jill, are sitting on the couch watching television. Suddenly Jeff stands and walks to the kitchen. What motivated his behavior? Jill could figure that out easily enough when her husband returned with a glass of water. Physical thirst. The body's need for fluid was communicated to the brain, and the sense of thirst motivated Jeff to search for water.

Jill cannot see "thirst," so in that sense it was hidden from her, but it was no less real. Most human behavior is motivated by what psychologists call the hidden self. Our motives are hidden from most observers and many close friends, even spouses. Behavior that is motivated by internal physical needs is probably the easiest to observe and understand. When we are having difficulty breathing, we will drop everything in search of air. When the body is too cold, we find ourselves searching for heat and when the body is too hot, we search for cool air. But behavior motivated by psychological or spiritual needs is much harder to recognize. Yet understanding such behavior—exposing the hidden self—is crucial for helping your spouse and your marriage.

For the individual who seeks to be a positive change agent in a troubled marriage, reality living must be coupled with one other important factor: understanding the motivation behind human behavior, both yours and that of your spouse. It's likely that your spouse's negative behavior has been a big part of your troubled marriage. Understanding the inner motivation behind your spouse's unreasonable, illogical, hurtful, and often destructive behavior may give you helpful insight as you seek to take a new approach to your life and marriage. Insight into *your own* inner self also may help, as you evaluate your own behavior more realistically.

Jill was fairly certain about the motive for Jeff's behavior, for it originated in the physical realm. Remember, though, motives are far less clear in the psychological realm, and most human behavior is motivated by psychological or spiritual needs. In addition, physical and psychological needs often are intertwined. If you're a member of my family and see me going for a drink of water, you may assume that I am thirsty. Instead, it may be my way of escaping an unpleasant conversation with my wife. If you meet me in the kitchen and ask me if I am thirsty, I may say, "No. I simply couldn't take another minute listening to that chatterbox. She was driving me crazy." In reality, there may be even a deeper motivation. Perhaps I felt intimidated by the situation in which I found myself. I am not mature enough or perhaps don't understand myself enough to admit that I went for water because I felt intimidated. Thus, I may not always understand my own inner motivations for what I do.

Then how can we possibly understand someone else's behavior? We can't—totally. But we can have educated guesses. What is important is to know that all of my spouse's behavior is motivated by internal desires or needs.

Psychiatrist William Glasser says, "Everything we do—good or bad, effective or ineffective, painful or pleasurable, crazy or sane, sick or well, drunk or sober—is to satisfy powerful forces within ourselves."[1] This is Glasser's way of saying that even inappropriate behavior is serving some function. In some distorted way, such behavior is meeting a psychological need. The closer we can come to understanding the internal motivation for our spouse's behavior, the better equipped we are to be agents of positive change. If we can help him/her meet those needs in a healthier manner, then we may well see our spouse's behavior change in a positive direction.

For example, Barry complained that the biggest trouble in his marriage was that his wife tried to control him. "She thinks that she is smarter than I am. It's her arrogant attitude that makes me so angry," he said. His wife Sheila's perspective was "Any time I disagree with him and share my opinion, he thinks I am trying to control him. I don't want to control him; I just want to be a part of the decision." This battle had gone on for years before Barry and Sheila came to my office. We explored the motivation behind Sheila's behavior. It took awhile but Barry did finally realize that indeed her motivation was not to control him but that she simply wanted to be partners with him—a wife rather than a child. She wanted him to have the benefit of her input on the topic of discussion. She was not trying to force him to agree with her; she simply wanted to sense that her ideas were important to him.

When Barry began to understand these motives, his entire response to Sheila's behavior changed. He no longer became defensive, angry, and argumentative. He even came to welcome her input. How did this influence Sheila's behavior? Her screaming and name-calling stopped. She no longer had to use such antics to get his attention.

This chapter will not offer an exhaustive list of the inner psychological and spiritual needs that motivate human behavior. Instead, I want to describe a few of the primary inner drives, needs, and desires that often motivate our behavior. I am using the words *needs, drives,* and *desires* as synonyms, all describing those inner compulsions that motivate us to take action. I am also using the words *psychological* and *spiritual* to describe those nonphysical needs that so profoundly affect our inner sense of well-being.

THE NEED FOR LOVE

First, and in my opinion most fundamental, is the need to love and be loved. I feel good about myself when I am helping others. This desire to love others accounts for the charitable, altruistic side of man. On the other hand, much of our behavior is motivated by the desire to receive love. I feel loved when I have the sense that people genuinely care for me, that my well-being is important to them, that they are genuinely looking out for my interests and giving of themselves for my well-being.

This kind of love is the opposite of loneliness. If I feel loved by my spouse, I have the sense of closeness or intimacy, but if I feel I've received little love—if my love tank is empty—I may feel cut off and alone. Much of my behavior, both positive and negative, is motivated by my need for love.

Joe is giving his wife tender, loving words. Why? Because he has learned from past experience that when he speaks kindly to her, she tends to reciprocate with loving words and acts toward him. His words are motivated at least in part by his own need for love. This does not deny his genuine concern for her well-being. If this exists, he is also meeting his need to give love.

Melanie, on the other hand, complains that her husband does not give her enough time. She often raises her voice and delivers angry lectures to him, accusing him of not caring for her. Why is Melanie involved in such negative behavior? It is her effort to try to meet her need for love. Perhaps it has been successful in the past. Perhaps it will be successful in the future, but almost everyone agrees that it is inappropriate and negative behavior. Thus much of our behavior, positive and negative, appropriate and inappropriate, is motivated by an effort to meet our need for love.

THE NEED FOR FREEDOM

Then there is the need for freedom—the desire to order my own life and not to be controlled by another. What we want is freedom to choose how we live our lives. In a marriage, we want to be free to express our feelings, thoughts, and desires. We want to be free to choose the goals that we will pursue. We want the freedom to read and write what satisfies us, to watch the TV programs in which we have an interest.

This desire for freedom is so strong that whenever we feel that our spouse is trying to manipulate or control us, we tend to become defensive and angry. Our sense of well-being about our marriage dissipates, and we have an awareness that our relationship is not healthy. Our marriage is not likely to return to a state of equilibrium as long as we have the sense that the other is trying to control us.

It will be obvious to most that the need for freedom and the need for love are often in conflict. This is why some men are hesitant to marry. They are wonderful lovers so long as their relationship is at the dating stage, but they are reluctant to make the commitment to marriage because they fear this will remove their freedom. A married man may move out of a marriage in search of freedom but soon finds himself lonely and seeking love. The couple who does not find the balance between love and freedom will never have a satisfying marriage. To find the balance between meeting these two needs requires give and take. We must give love and give freedom if we expect to receive love and freedom.

Freedom is never without boundaries. Freedom is never absolute; to be totally free is to live a life without love. If I am governed only by my own desires and give no consideration to others, I will soon be in bondage to my desires. Giving one's spouse freedom to choose to spend an evening watching a sports event or a dramatic production is far different from giving one's spouse freedom to have a relationship with a member of the opposite sex. The idea of "open marriage" which allows each to have intimate relationships with others has never proven to be a functional form of marriage for one simple reason. It violates true love. None of us wants our spouse to have that kind of freedom nor should we demand it for ourselves. On the other hand, none of us desires to be controlled in every area of life by our spouses. Such control also violates love.

Much of our behavior is motivated by our desire for freedom. Barry's defensive, angry outbursts at Sheila were motivated by his need for freedom. He perceived that Sheila was trying to control him; therefore, his angry behavior was designed to throw off that control and have freedom. When he realized that she was not in fact trying to control him, his angry outbursts ceased. He was no longer motivated to throw off her control because he no longer sensed that she was trying to control him.

When your spouse angrily accuses you of trying to control

his/her behavior, your partner is giving you a clue as to what motivates such inappropriate behavior—a need for freedom. Jordan has been encouraging his wife, Linda, to lose weight. He has said it often enough and strongly enough that she now feels that he is trying to control her. In addition, she feels that he does not love her as she is. One night, he again brings up the subject and she unloads her fiery cannon of flaming words, accusing him of not loving her and trying to control her.

What motivated nice, calm Linda to such explosive behavior? Maybe it was her need for love and her need for freedom. Did her behavior meet her needs? Perhaps, if thirty minutes later Jordan comes in, apologizes, verbally assures her of his love, tenderly embraces her, and assures her that it is not his desire to control her and if he doesn't mention her weight again for at least six months, then perhaps her angry behavior served to meet her need for love and freedom. Was her behavior positive, appropriate, constructive? The answer is no. Did it meet her needs? The answer is yes, at least momentarily. One of the tasks in a maturing marriage is to learn to meet our needs in a more mature and wholesome manner and to help our spouse discover the same.

THE NEED FOR SIGNIFICANCE

A third need that motivates much of our behavior is our need for significance. There is within each of us the desire to do something bigger than ourselves, to accomplish something that will impact the world, that will give us a sense of fulfillment and satisfaction. This need often motivates altruistic behavior. It is sometimes behind the driven nature of the workaholic. Much of human behavior is motivated by this desire to make a significant impact on the world, something for which we will be remembered.

Many times this drive for significance is heightened by childhood experiences. The father who tells his son that he will never amount to anything and for whom the efforts of his son are never quite enough influences the psychological perspective of his son, who may spend a lifetime trying to prove his father wrong and thus obtain significance. Understanding this motivation will greatly enhance the efforts of someone who is married to the workaholic.

More about this in a later chapter.

THE NEED FOR RECREATION

A fourth need is the need for recreation or relaxation. Physically, mentally, and emotionally, humans are designed with the need for rhythm, of movement between work and play. The old saying "All work and no play makes Jack a dull boy" reflects a fundamental need. This is readily observed by a candid look at our lifestyle. We invest much time and money in play. Take an inventory of the sports equipment in your own house and you will likely find an array of costly signs of this reality.

The men and women who play on the professional sports teams of our nation may be working, but the thousands who watch them are playing. They are unwinding from a stress-filled week. They are enjoying a time with friends; they are socializing, laughing, and relaxing. They are avid in their desire to have fun.

Look at your own behavior and the behavior of your spouse and you will see at least some of your behavior is motivated by this desire for recreation and relaxation. The methods of meeting this need are myriad and are colored by our unique preferences, but all of us look forward to the fun times of life in which we can relax and enjoy the things and relationships which we have accumulated. Why does Bill come home, click on the TV, and enjoy his favorite drink before engaging in conversation with his wife, Tess? Because he wants to relax before he is faced with the stress of relating to her. Consciously or unconsciously, he is seeking to meet his need for relaxation.

Tess may interpret this behavior as lack of love for her, but if she understands his motivation perhaps she can find a way to get the love she needs and still allow him the freedom to meet his own needs. She too must find her own way of relaxing, or she will lose her inner psychological equilibrium.

THE NEED FOR PEACE WITH GOD

Then there is what I call the need for peace with God. This is at the center of man's inner self. The thousands of volumes that deal with religious and spiritual issues testify to the depth of this need. Modern man may have rejected organized religion, but modern man has not abandoned his search for spiritual reality. The avowed atheist will be found on occasion calling the TV psychic line, or after midnight, watching the TV evangelist or sitting in a silent corner reading the writings of some ancient or modern mystic. There is something within man that reaches out to make connection with the nonphysical world. This need for a spiritual connection has not been eradicated by modern scientific dogmas and much of human behavior is motivated by this search for peace with God.

Traci was incredulous at her husband Todd's recent interest in studying the Bible. She said to me with fire in her eyes, "I don't understand this and I don't like it. He spends two or three nights a week reading the Bible and working through a study guide given to him by a friend. He has even asked me to attend the Bible study with him. This is a man who has been an atheist since the tenth grade. In college, he made fun of Christians and often took pleasure in debating them. He assured me before we got married that religion would never be a part of our lives and now he is becoming a fundamentalist Bible freak. Explain that to me."

I didn't sense that Traci was open to an explanation at that moment, and I was deeply sympathetic with her frustration at this sudden turn of events in her husband. But I was certain that Todd was on a search for peace with God. His behavior was motivated by his inner need for a spiritual dimension to his life.

Philosophers and world leaders have always seen man as possessing a nonmaterial dimension. Blaise Pascal, the French philosopher said, "The most important thought that ever occupied my mind is that of my individual responsibility to God." Abraham Lincoln noted, "It is difficult to make a man miserable while he feels he is worthy of himself and claims kindred to the great God who made him." Dag Hammarskjold, former secretary-general of the United Nations said, "God does not die on the day when we cease to believe in a personal deity, but we die on the day when our lives cease to be illuminated by the steady radiance, renewed daily, of a wonder, the source of which is beyond all reason."[2] Man has a spiritual hunger that impels him to seek meaning beyond the world of food, sex, and activities. Man has a need to find peace with God.

DISCOVERING MOTIVES

These are examples of the kind of inner psychological-spiritual needs that motivate much of human behavior. People do not climb mountains because they are there; they climb for freedom, fun, companionship, significance, or to find solitude—but not to find out what's on top. If we are to understand each other, we must ask the questions: "What motivates my spouse's behavior? What needs is he/she consciously or subconsciously trying to meet? What motivates my own behavior? What needs am I trying to meet?" As we answer those questions we are more able to understand human behavior.

Your method for discovering motivations may involve studying books on human nature which explore man's basic needs, some of which we have touched upon in this chapter. It may involve overtly asking questions of your spouse. Looking at your own inner motivations may give you clues as to what is behind your spouse's behavior. Hopefully as you read the illustrations in this book, you will be able to see parallels in your marriage. None of these approaches will give exact answers, but all may help you make an educated guess about the motivation behind your spouse's troublesome behavior. It is understanding this inner motivation that enlightens you to take actions designed to stimulate constructive change in your spouse's behavior.

RECOGNIZING FOUR TYPES OF PERSONALITY

One other aspect of the hidden self greatly impacts our behavior. It is what we typically call *personality,* our patterned way of responding to life. When people speak of others as *extroverted* or *introverted, neat* or *sloppy, pessimistic* or *optimistic, decisive* or *indecisive, excitable* or *calm,* they are talking about personality traits. They are predictable ways in which one tends to respond to life's situations.

Marlene said of her husband, Josh, "He is so slow and deliberate that by the time he makes a decision, it is too late." Marlene is talking about one of Josh's personality traits. We all have a mixture of these personality characteristics, and someone who knows us well can usually predict how we will respond in a given situation. There are scores of these personality traits, and they tend to cluster in certain patterns. Thus, we speak of personality types. There are various personality inventories which, if taken, will reveal one's pattern of personality traits. If you and your spouse have never taken such a personality test, it can be both an enjoyable and insightful experience. Such tests are easily arranged through a local counselor's office.

It is beyond the scope of this chapter to exhaustively explore personality. But let me mention four common types as illustrative of the importance of understanding personality if we are to understand the hidden self. First is *the peacemaker*. This is the calm, slow, easy-going, well-balanced personality. This person is typically pleasant, doesn't like conflicts, seldom seems ruffled, and rarely expresses anger.

The peacemaker has emotions, but does not easily reveal them. In a marriage and family setting, the peacemaker wants calm, tends to ignore conflicts, and avoids arguments at all costs. This leads to the tendency to leave conflicts unresolved. If the argument does break out, the peacemaker will seek to calm the other person by acquiescing even if he does not fully agree. He is kindhearted and sympathetic and wants everybody just to enjoy life. The peacemaker is typically easy to live with, but his low-pressure way of life may be a source of irritation. Peacemakers make good companions to their children and tend to be contented spouses so long as there are no major conflicts in the relationship.

The second personality type is *the controller*. The controller is the quick, active, practical, strong-willed person. She tends to be self-sufficient, independent, decisive, and opinionated. Finding it easy to make decisions for herself, she often makes decisions for other people as well.

The controller thrives on activity. Her mind is constantly filled with ideas, plans, and ambitions. The controller will take definite stands on issues and can often be found crusading for her (or his) special cause. She does not give in to the pressure of others but will argue to the end, always winning. Problems are seen as challenges to the controller. She has dogged determination and does not sympathize easily with others. The controller does not easily express compassion or warm emotions. Though controllers are well-organized in their thinking, they tend to see the overall picture rather than the details. Once they have set their goal, they often run over individuals who stand in their way.

Then there is *the caretaker*. This is the self-sacrificing, gifted perfectionist who wants to meet the needs of others. His emotional nature is extremely sensitive. He often expresses feelings of gloom and depression because he sees the pain and hurts of the world. The caretaker is extremely dependable and has high standards for himself as well as others. The caretaker often has exceptional analytical abilities and is able to see the pitfalls in reaching a goal; thus, often he throws cold water on the controller's ideas.

The caretaker finds his/her greatest meaning in life through personal sacrifice and service to others. They will be persistent in their pursuit of doing good. The downside of this personality type is that they often burn themselves out and fail to recognize their own emotional needs.

Finally, there is *the party maker*. This is the warm, lively, excited personality. For this person, all of life is a party. The party maker enjoys people, does not like solitude, and is at her best when surrounded by friends where she is usually "the life of the party." The party maker makes life exciting not only for herself but for others. Filled with stories, dramatic expressions, and song, the party maker's objective is that everyone should be happy.

Party makers are never at a loss for words; they are always busy either attending parties or getting ready for parties. A simple meal is a celebration. The downside of this personality is that people with this personality type come across as undependable and undisciplined. They are so much into the moment that they often forget previous commitments.

Each of these personality patterns has strengths and weaknesses when it comes to the marital relationship. Although none of us fits neatly into these four personality patterns, we all tend to identify with one more than the others. Seldom do a husband and wife have the same personality. We tend to be attracted to those who have opposite traits from our own. We are attracted to those who have strengths in the areas where we are weak. These differences, however, often tend to annoy us once we are married.

Personality patterns do not greatly change once they are established. Whether they are hereditary or learned in early childhood is inconsequential. This is not to say that we cannot have significant growth in the weak areas of our personality. It does mean that we will always have the natural tendency to behave in keeping with our basic personality.

Personality Interactions Between Husbands and Wives

The important thing is understanding your own personality and that of your spouse. The reason that it is so important to understand personality patterns is that we tend to seek to meet our psychological and spiritual needs in keeping with our personality. For example, the caretaker, in seeking to meet her need for significance, will often find herself enmeshed in caring for a needy friend. She will spend hours trying to help this friend solve problems and find meaning to life. However, the efforts of the caretaker will often be incomprehensible to the controller. "Why would anyone spend so much time and energy trying to help such a loser?" is the attitude of the controller. The controller fails to recognize that the caretaker is finding her own significance in caring for the needy person. It is her way of meeting one of her deepest inner needs—the need for significance. The controller, on the other hand, would typically meet his need for significance by building a great organization, building, or business.

The caretaker may be critical of the controller's strong, dominating determination, which may be hurting people in the process of reaching his goals. But if the caretaker understands that reaching the goal is the controller's effort to meet his need for significance, she will better understand his behavior. Perhaps she will decide to help the people he is hurting and thus, both of them are meeting their need for significance.

The methods we use to satisfy our hidden need to love and be loved, our need for freedom, significance, recreation or relaxation, peace with God, and all other psychological and spiritual needs will be influenced by our personality. Understanding this reality will give you significant insight into your own behavior and that of your spouse. In fact, the manner in which you seek to be a positive change agent in your marriage will be greatly influenced by your personality.

Your efforts in the past have also been influenced by your personality. For example, if you are a peacemaker, you have probably tried to overlook the things about your spouse that have irritated or disappointed you. You have not been quick to argue but by nature have held your pain inside. Such behavior, which is your natural pattern, can lead to great emotional distance between you and your spouse. When the distance becomes unbearable, you will tend to go against your personality and try a different approach. This is often necessary. However, the first step is understanding your own personality and why you have taken the approach you have taken in the past. Remember, we are influenced by our personality but we are not controlled by our personality. When we see a better way, we must be willing to take it even though it takes us outside our comfort zone.

In the following chapters, we will seek to apply the principles discussed in these first five chapters. We will look at how reality living, understanding motives, and recognizing personality types can help us deal more effectively with our spouses. I will take you behind closed doors, as we look at married couples (whose identities have all been disguised) and explore the characteristics of various troubled marriages. We will examine the actions that other husbands and wives have taken based upon reality living and the results they have experienced.

None of these stories will exactly match your own, but hopefully they will be close enough to give you insights and ideas on positive steps which you may take in seeking to stimulate positive change in your marital relationship.

NOTES

1. William Glasser, *Control Theory: A New Explanation of How We Control Our Lives* (New York: Perennial, 1985), 2.
2. George Sweeting, *Who Said That?* (Chicago: Moody, 1994), 209, 304.

THE IRRESPONSIBLE
SPOUSE

When we enter marriage, we assume we are marrying a responsible person. We assume that he will carry his part of the load. We know that our roles will be somewhat different, but we each assume that our spouse will use his mind, skills, and energy for our mutual benefit. When it seems apparent that our spouse is not the responsible person we thought we married, we feel hurt, angry, and often agitated.

Our response to an irresponsible spouse will vary depending upon our own personality. If we are by nature a "controller," we will likely deliver angry lectures about her irresponsibility. We may accuse her of being lazy like her mother or father. Or we may accuse her of being a spoiled brat whose parents did everything for her and now she expects us to do the same. If, on the other hand we are by nature peacemakers, we may suffer in silence rather than draw attention to our spouse's irresponsible behavior and create an argument. Whatever our response, we will be pained and frustrated by our spouse's behavior. "It's just not fair," we may think. "I work hard. Why can't she?" Or we may reason, "I don't think I'm expecting too much. I just want him to be responsible." If our spouse's irresponsible behavior continues over a long period of time, we will indeed find ourselves in a troubled marriage.

For the ten years of Elaine and Bill's marriage, the longest time Bill had held a job was eighteen months. In chapter 1 we met Elaine, upset about her husband Bill's irresponsible employment history.

Bill's job problems varied. Sometimes, he would get in a fight with a fellow employee and simply walk off the job. Other times, he would get frustrated with the job or the people with whom he worked and simply go home one evening and never return. Between jobs, he would often go weeks and sometimes months without work. He spent his time sleeping late, watching television, and working out at the local gym. On the other hand, Elaine had worked a full-time job all ten years of their marriage, except for brief times surrounding the births of their two children. When Bill had a job, he would help Elaine with the bills but when he was out of work, she had to carry the whole load.

The tears were flowing freely when Elaine said, "Dr. Chapman, I don't know how much longer I can go on like this." Elaine was living with an irresponsible husband and she was deeply troubled.

Like Elaine, Becky also had a troubled marriage, but unemployment was not the issue. Both David and she held full-time jobs while rearing three children during their fifteen years of marriage. Her complaint was David's passive lifestyle. "He takes no initiative to do anything except to work regularly. Our bedroom has needed painting for six years. Over and over he says, 'I'll get around to it,' but he never has. The children's bicycles stay broken for months before he finally gets around to fixing them. Our money sits in a passbook savings account and he will take no initiative to try to discover an investment where we can get a better return. In the summer, the grass gets mowed every three weeks. I'm ashamed to have my friends come by. In fact, last summer I finally hired someone to mow the grass every week.

"He spends his time with his computer. Everyone talks about how great computers are; actually I hate them. I wish the thing would just explode and he would wake up in the real world. I've tried everything I know. I've tried calmly discussing the matter with him, I've tried screaming at him, I've tried ignoring the problem, I've tried being overly kind to him. Nothing seems to make a difference. I don't know what else to do."

Elaine and Becky have very different husbands, but they are both complaining about their husbands' lack of assertiveness in facing life. The files of counselors are filled with records of wives' complaining about husbands who have no ambition. But there are also husbands who have similar complaints about their wives.

Robert waited until he was thirty-nine before he married. He prided himself on being a bachelor. However, Suzanne swept him off his feet. The top salesperson in her company for the past two years, she was attractive, playful, and deeply in love with Robert. She also had a five-year-old daughter by a previous marriage. Robert was her ideal man. She had dreamed of marrying a man who wanted a stay-at-home wife. She wanted to leave the workforce and devote her energies to raising her child. She also hoped to have other children. Robert was her man, they both agreed.

The first year of marriage was wonderful. Suzanne continued to work so that they could get the house and furniture they both wanted. And by the end of the year, they both agreed it was time for her to quit work. They were both excited about reaching this goal, but that is when the problems started. Seven years later, I met a very frustrated husband. Robert complained that when he arrived home in the afternoon, he had to shovel his way through the house. He could not imagine how the house could be in such disarray in one day or why Suzanne could not arrange to have things "in order" before he arrived home. His other complaint was that Suzanne did not cook dinner for him. She fed the children, but most of the time he had to find his own food.

"Sometimes, I have to turn around and go to the grocery store after I get home from work. I don't understand why she can't keep at least the basics in the house," he said.

"I was happy for her to quit work. I knew that was something she wanted to do, but I thought that if she were going to stay at home, she would at least keep the house clean and cook dinner for me. I don't mind going out one or two evenings a week, but she seems to have no concern and senses no responsibility for fixing dinner or keeping the house in order." He had complained and given lectures for years, but Suzanne had not changed. In Robert's mind, he was married to an irresponsible wife. Her irresponsibility was a barrier to marital intimacy.

Elaine, Becky, and Robert were each frustrated, hurt, angry, resentful, and miserable. They each felt that they had tried, really tried to work out their marital problems. They realized that their efforts had not always been positive and that in fact sometimes, their efforts had compounded the problem. But they each were sincere in their efforts. When they arrived in my office, they had little hope. Their emotions said "Get out." Some of their friends had the same recommendation, but for various reasons, they did not want to give up on their marriage. Let me share with you the approach we took in helping them become positive change agents when seemingly irresponsible behaviors threatened their troubled marriages.

CLARIFYING THE PROBLEM

If we are to become positive change agents, we must first clarify the problem. Let's make sure that the problem really is lack of responsibility. Elaine, Becky, and Robert all complained that their spouses were irresponsible. Was this really the case? Our perception of reality is always colored by our own personality, values, and desires. Sometimes what we perceive is not objective reality. I remember the wife who complained that her husband had no ambition. In further conversation, I discovered that he held two full-time jobs and one part-time job. What did she mean, "no ambition"? She was a deeply religious woman, and her complaint was that he never took any initiative to read the Bible to the family and that he didn't do anything around the house. In her mind, he was an irresponsible husband. In reality, his problem was not lack of ambition. The problem was that all of his ambition was focused in one area—making money. His wife, who we will call Sally, desired that he be the spiritual leader in the home and give her practical help around the house. Sally was verbalizing that he had no ambition; in reality, he was a very ambitious husband. Thus, the answer lay not in trying to stimulate ambition but in helping him redirect his ambition into the areas that were important to his wife.

In further conversation, I found out that he had grown up in a poor family, and as a child he had determined that when he was an adult he would work hard and provide his family with the things he never had. In addition to his childhood experience, in the early days of their marriage, Sally had complained much about the finances. Again, he determined "to make the money." He was not a highly skilled man and in his mind the best way to secure the money was to work multiple jobs. Her complaints about him being irresponsible were totally incomprehensible to him.

Sally was, in fact, focusing her attention on the wrong problem. What she was calling irresponsibility was really a need for balance. With two full-time jobs and one part-time job, he was highly responsible in one area of the marriage—finances—but was neglecting responsibility in another—time with the family.

Now let's consider Becky, and David's supposed irresponsibility. David did not have multiple jobs, but he did have one very responsible job and was a good provider for the family. Becky's concern was that he took no initiative in other areas of the marriage. The unpainted bedroom, the children's broken bicycles, the passbook savings account, and the grass in the yard all cried for his attention while he devoted his time away from the job to his computer. He was not irresponsible in all areas of life, only in the areas of unpainted bedrooms, broken bicycles, savings crying for investment, and yard work—all of which were important to Becky.

Robert's wife, Suzanne, was also an extremely responsible person in one area—mothering. She loved being a stay-at-home mom and spent hours with her two children. She could have gotten the "Creative Mother of the Year" award for the kind of educational experiences she gave her children. She had demonstrated her ambition before marriage by being the number one salesperson for her company. Now she was turning her energies toward parenting. Keeping the house "in order" was not high on her priority list, although she did work at making the house safe for the children. She took care of the children's meals; but when it came to Robert, she thought, *Robert's an adult, and his schedule is unpredictable. He can take care of himself.* She could not understand Robert's concern. "We had agreed that I would quit work to take care of the children," she said. "I think I'm doing a good job. Why is he upset and why is he calling me irresponsible?"

Elaine, on the other hand, was married to a husband who was basically irresponsible in all areas of life. He did not maintain a regular job and thus did not carry his load in financial provision nor did he help around the house or spend much time with their two children. Bill was not carrying his part of the load in any area of life.

It is helpful to clarify the problem. It should be obvious that Elaine's problem with Bill is quite different from Becky's problem with David and Robert's problem with Suzanne. Thus their actions, designed to stimulate positive change, will need to be different.

ANALYZE THE SOURCE OF THE PROBLEM

It always helps to understand something of what is going on in the mind of your spouse. You are not likely to take the right actions without this insight. Let's assume that your husband really has little ambition. He won't work in the home or out of the home, or perhaps he has a regular job to which he is faithful but will do nothing but watch TV or play golf. He shows no interest in fathering or being a husband. What lies behind this seeming lack of ambition? Understanding the source of his behavior is a part of finding the cure. Let me suggest four possible sources.

First, he may be *following the model of his father.* Look at his father's lifestyle. Is he simply doing what he learned from his father? All of us are influenced by the model of our parents. Many men enter marriage and simply repeat the husband/father style which they have observed in their own father.

On the other hand, he may be *rebelling against the model of his father.* His father was a workaholic; he was never there for his son. His mother often complained about his father's work. So, as a young man, the husband decided that work was bad and that he would never repeat his father's mistake. Therefore, he is rebelling against his father's model. Many of us are keenly aware of our parents' failures. Some of us consciously or subconsciously are trying hard to be different. We do not want to repeat the mistakes of our parents. Often these efforts lead us to the other extreme. The son of a workaholic father may become irresponsible in his work patterns. The daughter of a promiscuous mother may become rigid in her attitudes toward sex.

A third possibility is that your husband *may have developed a self-centered attitude*. At the root of many unambitious spouses is pure and simple selfishness. Perhaps he was given few responsibilities growing up. His parents pampered him. He developed the mind-set of "everything comes to him who waits." He believes that the world owes him a living and sooner or later, the world will deliver. This person is a taker but not a giver. He has never learned to provide for others. His life has centered in others providing for him.

Fourth, your husband's behavior *may be an expression of his resentment toward you*. Whatever you want, he will lean in the opposite direction. If you are asking him to do things around the house, he will put them off because in his mind you do not deserve his help. He will likely see your requests as nagging or criticism. His only assertiveness is in making sure that he does not do what you request. In some area of life, he does not feel that you are meeting his needs. His lack of responsibility toward you is designed to draw attention to his own unmet needs.

These are not the only possibilities, but they are four common sources of irresponsibility. As you look for the source of your spouse's irresponsibility, it is helpful to remember that much of our behavior is motivated by our inner emotional needs, which we discussed in chapter 5. Remember, the most basic of those needs are for love, freedom, significance, recreation, and peace with God. The clearer you can understand the source of your spouse's behavior, the more likely you are to determine positive steps that you can take to stimulate constructive change.

Let's consider the source of Bill's irresponsible behavior. In further conversations with Elaine, I discovered that Bill was suffering from a severe case of insecurity and low self-esteem. He grew up with an alcoholic father who often told him that he would never amount to anything, who regularly criticized him and put down his efforts. Bill had shared all of this with Elaine when they were dating. He was attracted to her because she gave him positive affirmation. She told him how wrong his father was. Finally, Bill had met someone who believed in him and loved him. He responded by doing things that pleased Elaine. He sent her flowers and cards, something she had always associated with love. It is not hard to understand how the two of them could have fallen in love.

Bill had a job when they were married. He had been working there for the entire year that Elaine had known him. She had no way of knowing before the wedding that during the first ten years of their marriage his employment record would be so erratic; nor did she understand that Bill was filled with anger for his father. He was determined to prove his father wrong, but his anger led him to sharp words and critical comments to fellow employees. When they responded in like manner, Bill's self-esteem was threatened. They were giving him the same message his father had given him, and so he would leave the job.

The first time he left the job, Elaine was supportive and verbally affirmed him. He felt her love and sought diligently for a second job. When that job lasted only six months, Elaine was not as supportive but rather questioned him about why he had to leave this job. From that juncture, her comments to him about each successive job loss became more critical. Elaine was no longer his source of love and security. She had joined the voice of his father in condemning him. He had, in fact, come to believe the message. He was no good; he was a loser. Soon Bill was suffering from depression.

The source of his irresponsible behavior was that his need for significance was not being met, and the love which he had received from Elaine had now dried up. His employment record and his depressed behavior of sleeping late and watching television were his cries for self-esteem and love, but that is not what Elaine saw. What she saw was his irresponsible behavior, and what she felt was lack of love. Her own need for love and support was not met, and her response had been to criticize Bill for his irresponsibility. Understanding the source of Bill's behavior made it possible for Elaine to take positive steps to influence his behavior.

Becky discovered something quite different in her husband, David. He was very successful in his job and was encouraged because the rewards from hard work fed his self-esteem. But his need for love was not being met in the marriage. His response was to draw back from his wife. His primary love language was *words of affirmation*. But increasingly he heard criticism about spending so much time with his computer (which was his way of relaxing) and doing so little to help her and the children. It seemed to him that Becky seldom gave him a positive word. His love tank was empty, and his irresponsible behavior was shouting, "I will not respond to the requests of one who is not loving me." His irresponsible behavior did not engender love feelings or actions from Becky.

Thus, the trouble in their relationship had compounded over the years. When Becky began to understand what was happening inside David, she began to get a new perspective on how she could become a change agent in their marriage.

When Robert began to focus on the source of Suzanne's behavior, he discovered that she still had a lot of guilt over taking her daughter through a divorce. Before her marriage to Robert, she had focused her attention on her daughter. She was excelling in her sales job, but with all of her free time she was seeking to enrich her daughter's life. After she was able to become a stay-at-home mom and after she and Robert had their own child, she was even more determined to be a good mother.

By the time she had married Robert, her sense of self-worth was strong. She had been a successful career woman. She was now ready to succeed in another area—parenting. Robert's well-paying vocation enabled her to do this. She was well on her way until Robert started complaining about her housekeeping and not cooking meals. She felt he was being unfair and was failing to recognize the value of her spending time with the children. When his complaints continued, she felt he was trying to control her life. He was trying to steal her freedom. She refused to buckle to his demands and resolved that neither he nor anyone else would keep her from investing time with her children. He was no longer affirming her self-worth, and in time she was feeling unloved by Robert. This made it even more difficult for her to be responsive to his demands. This insight set Robert on a whole new course of action, which brings us to the third and most important consideration.

TAKE POSITIVE ACTION

Robert was now ready to take action, applying the principles of reality living. He realized that he was responsible for his own attitude. He could think positive in spite of the negative factors in his marriage. If he looked for the positive, he would find it. He discovered that attitudes affect actions, that if he chose to believe there were solutions, he would seek those solutions and take positive steps in the right direction. Although he could not change Suzanne's behavior, Robert understood that he could influence her by his positive actions. He realized that he could take such actions even while his emotions were negative.

Robert also knew that he had made many mistakes in his efforts to change Suzanne. He was now willing to admit those mistakes and realized that in so doing, he was not admitting that he was a failure nor was he taking all the blame for their problems.

He also discovered that love is the most powerful weapon for good in the world. He began to ask himself, "What loving actions can I take toward Suzanne that have the potential for influencing her in a positive way?" Here are the actions that Robert took.

He began by *acknowledging his own imperfections*. He was not certain that he could verbalize his thoughts to Suzanne, so he decided to write her a letter. His letter went something like this:

Dear Suzanne,

I have been thinking about us for the past few days. I realize that for a long time, I have been overly critical of you. I know that my criticism must have hurt you deeply. I want you to know that I realize that I have been wrong and I want to ask you to forgive me for all of my critical and demanding lectures.

When we got married, I was proud of you for your accomplishments in the business world. I know now that I should be proud of you for all that you are doing for our children. I don't think there could be a better mother. I guess I have just felt left out of your love and maybe that's why I have been so critical. That doesn't excuse it; I am just trying to understand my own behavior. I know that you probably have not felt much love from me either. I think we both need and deserve more from each other.

I know that I want to make the future different. I want to feel close to you again, and I want to join you in parenting. I know that I have a lot to learn about being a father, but I want to be what my children need. I am open to your suggestions on how I can be a better husband and a better father. I hope you can tell by the tenor of this letter that I am sincere. Whenever you have had a chance to read this, maybe we can talk about it. I love you very much.

Robert

The letter was hard to write; the words did not come easy. But Robert knew that he was taking a different approach, and he sensed that he was on the right track. You will note that in his letter his comments were based upon Suzanne's need for freedom and love. He also expressed his own need to receive love from her.

Second, *he expressed his love to her.* He gave her words of affirmation about her mothering skills, words which he had not spoken in many months. A week later, they did discuss the letter, and he was able to affirm verbally his love for her.

Third, *he asked for suggestions* on how to be a better husband and father. Robert asked if she would give him one suggestion every two weeks; he knew that he could not change everything all at once, but he thought this might be a good way to get started. Suzanne agreed that if he were sincere she would be willing to make such suggestions. Her first suggestion was that when he came home at night, rather than making comments about the house, he should find each of the children, give them a big hug, and spend a few minutes of quality time with each child. Then she wanted him to find her, give her a hug and kiss, and they would spend five minutes sharing with each other the kind of day they had. Robert was willing to take this step and, in fact, seldom missed a day.

Suzanne continued to give a suggestion every two weeks, and he continued to respond. After two months, he asked Suzanne "How do you think I am doing in my efforts to be a better husband and father?" She overwhelmed him with her answer. "I could not be happier with all the changes you have made. I think I have died and gone to heaven." Robert had to admit that her response gave him warm feelings toward her. It had been a long time since he had heard such affirming words.

SLOW, STEADY CHANGE

Suzanne's behavior did not change immediately. In fact, Robert saw only slight changes in her behavior toward him. There were a few times that she cooked a good meal and the family ate together. Robert told her what a good cook she was and how much he enjoyed the meal. He succeeded in not adding his usual comment, "I wish you would do this more often." Robert continued to take Suzanne's suggestions seriously. Most of the things she requested he was able to do. He started giving the children a bath once a week. On Saturdays, he would keep the children for two hours while Suzanne played volleyball with friends. Later, as the children got older, he would sometimes take them to watch her play.

Four months into Robert's new approach, he made his first request of Suzanne. One night he said, "Would you like to do something that would make me really happy?" to which she responded, "I might." "You know those wonderful apple pies you used to make when we were first married? I love your apple pies. Would it be possible for you to make an apple pie some time this week or next?" She smiled and said, "Do they still make apples?" In less than a week, Robert had his homemade apple pie. Not only did he tell her how wonderful it was, but the next week when they were with friends he announced, "Suzanne's apple pie would win a blue ribbon at the fair. You wouldn't believe her crust."

Before six months had rolled around, Suzanne had decided that she would like to start receiving a suggestion from Robert every two weeks on how she could be a better wife, things that would please him. Robert could not believe his ears, but he was willing to comply with her request.

Over the next six months, both of them continued to give suggestions to each other, and each of them continued to make constructive changes. Before the year was out, Suzanne was tutoring a neighbor high school student in business math for an hour each afternoon in exchange for the girl watching the children for forty-five minutes while Suzanne "got the house in order for Robert." Robert was shocked when he walked into the house the first afternoon. After three days of this, he knew something was up, so he asked Suzanne what was going on. She told him about her tutoring plan. Robert was incredulous that she would go to that much trouble to do something that he had not yet been bold enough to request. She was also cooking the evening meal Monday, Wednesday, and Friday nights; Tuesday and Thursday they were going out to eat and Saturday and Sunday were free-for-all. Suzanne had indeed changed.

What stimulated this positive change in her behavior? Robert's understanding of her inner needs and a willingness to change his own behavior. He backed off from seeking to control her behavior, thus giving her freedom. He began to give her affirming words for her mothering skills, which built her self-esteem and sense of significance. He began to express love in ways that she requested, giving himself to make life easier for her. She could now respond to his requests because she no longer felt that he was trying to control her. Her sense of significance and worth was returning because he was affirming her. She was feeling loved by him because he responded to her requests; thus she was able to reciprocate his love.

All of this happened a number of years ago. Robert and Suzanne continue to have a strong, growing, supportive marriage. But when I first encountered Robert, he had no hope that his marriage could ever be this wonderful. He is one of many who discovered that reality living can bring hope into what seems to be a hopeless situation.

Becky's story is very similar. She applied the same principles and took basically the same steps that Robert took. When she realized that David's behavior found its root in his need for significance and self-worth and that his resentment of her was growing out of his need for love, she realized that her negative pattern had been compounding the problem. When she further realized that his language of love was words of affirmation, she more deeply understood why he had withdrawn from her. She had given him exactly the opposite—complaining, condemning words. She understood more fully how her condemning words had pushed him to his computer.

ASKING FORGIVENESS

One night Becky apologized for her critical comments and asked David's forgiveness. She explained how feelings of deep frustration had been allowed to control her behavior.

"I have decided that I am going to focus on changing my negative behavior and try to make life more pleasant for you in the future. I am open to your suggestions in how I can do this." And she lauded David: "You are a hardworking man, and you have accomplished many things in your vocation. Most women would be proud of your accomplishments, but I have been extremely critical of you because you have not done the things that I wanted. I realize how selfish I have been."

David's response went something like this: "I never thought I would hear you say that. I thought I was the worst person in the world in your mind. I admit that I have had a lot of resentment toward you. I have not felt that you loved me for a long time and that you were trying to control my life. I was determined not to let that happen. I guess we both need to make some changes."

A week later, Becky asked for David's suggestion on one thing she could do to make life easier for him. That first night, David did something that I have seldom seen happen—he said he would give her such a suggestion if she would also give him one. This set in motion a process that changed both of their lives. When a marriage has been troubled for many years, such reciprocal openness is not the norm. Robert's experience of going several months with little response is a much more typical pattern. For some reason, David was so impressed with the sincerity of Becky's approach that he reciprocated much more quickly than most.

Two years after Becky's new beginning, she was taking a computer course at the local technical institute. David painted the bedroom within the first six months, and when summer rolled around he never missed a week at mowing the grass. In Becky's words, "He became a totally different man. I can't believe we went so long in such misery and that things turned around so quickly."

On the other hand, Elaine has not had such miraculous results, although she has seen positive change. Unlike Robert and Becky, Elaine was dealing with a different kind of irresponsibility. Her husband Bill was basically irresponsible in *all* areas of life. He would not maintain a regular job, would not help her around the house, was not involved in parenting their two children, and essentially did only what he desired to do. For ten years, Elaine had carried the load financially and in all other areas of the marriage.

By the time I saw Elaine, Bill was suffering from deep depression and spent the bulk of his time sleeping, watching television, and working out at the local gym. Bill was suffering from insecurity and low self-esteem. He was living out the message he had received from his alcoholic father that he was worthless and that he would never amount to anything. His anger for his father that he had exhibited toward fellow employees remained, a key reason he had never been able to hold a steady job. Bill did not feel loved by Elaine, and in his heart he felt that he did not deserve her love. He knew that he had failed her as a husband and often wondered why she put up with him.

All of these realities had to be considered in Elaine's approach at trying to be a positive change agent in her troubled marriage. Remembering that Bill had responded well to her words of encouragement and affirmation in their dating relationship and in the first year of their marriage, and realizing that she had been giving him critical words for the last nine years, she decided to begin by acknowledging what she considered to be her major failure.

"I've been thinking a lot about us and I have realized that for the past several years, I have helped compound your problems by being critical of you. I know that my critical words have not helped you," she began. "I want you to know that I still love you even though I am sure that you haven't felt much love from me over the past few years.

LOVING SOLUTIONS

A TIME FOR TOUGH LOVE

"I must confess that I have been deeply disappointed with our marriage, and I do not wish to continue as we are. I know that a part of your problem is your depression, and I know that life has not been easy for you. I have decided that I will be willing to pay for your counseling if you would be willing to go. This is the only hope I see for your getting help and for our marriage getting better. If you are not willing to go for counseling, then I cannot remain in the marriage, even though I love you very much. If you are willing to go for counseling, I have a suggestion of a good counselor. He is one I can afford and I think he will be able to help you. I want you to think about it and let me know your decision tomorrow."

Bill didn't say anything. So after a moment of silence, Elaine turned and walked out of the room. The next night, Bill was not there. He did not return in time for supper, which was not unusual. About 8:30 P.M. he came into the house, sat down on the couch, and flipped on the TV as was his habit. After Elaine got the children to bed, she waited until the TV program Bill was watching had ended. She walked into the room, flipped off the TV and said, "I can't tell you how much I love you and I hope you know that I would not be doing what I am doing if I didn't really care about you and about us. I need to know your decision. Do you want to see a counselor or do you want to call our marriage quits?"

"I want to see a counselor," he said. "I know I've got problems and I'm not getting any better. I don't know how you've put up with me this long."

"I'm glad," she said. "It's the only hope I see for either one of us." She reached for her purse and handed him the name of a counselor with a telephone number. "Here's the counselor I think you should see. Tomorrow, I want you to call and make an appointment. I've already checked. My insurance will pay for part of it, and I will take care of the rest until you get better and can get a job. Bill, I don't care how long it takes. I just want to see things different for you and for us."

The next day, Bill called the counselor, and the next week he began the long process of dealing with his current depression, his

84

long-term anger toward his father, and his learned patterns of irresponsibility. Within three months, Bill was looking for another job and within three weeks, he found one. He continued his counseling for two years. The counselor was able to help Bill understand why he had lost his temper so often on the job, how he had transferred his anger with his father toward fellow employees. Eventually, he learned how to release his anger toward his father; he found inner healing, and today he and his father have a cordial relationship.

More importantly, Bill learned how to process his anger on the job and at home. He and Elaine are in the process of building a meaningful marriage. They are still strapped with financial debt from the past, but for the first time, Elaine believes that soon they will be able to deal with the debt. She has given Bill affirming words throughout the years of his recovery. He is slowly learning how to be a father to his children and how to express love to Elaine on an emotional level. He acknowledges that it has been a long road, but he is encouraged by the progress he has seen. They both know that the journey is not over, but for the first time in ten years they both believe that they are on a positive track.

Elaine's application of reality living required very different actions from Robert and Becky because the inner motivation of Bill's irresponsible behavior was vastly different from that of David and Suzanne. If we are to be constructive change agents toward irresponsible spouses, we must always consider what motivates their irresponsible behavior, what is going on inside the individual. Unless we are able to address these issues, we are not likely to see positive change.

Sometimes, as in the case of Elaine, our efforts must be geared toward getting the spouse to a counselor. The problem is so severe that neither spouse will be able to handle it alone. Other times, as in the case of Robert and Becky, our efforts are designed at identifying the role our own behavior has played in compounding the problem of irresponsibility in our spouse and taking steps to meet the inner needs for love, self-worth, and significance. Always there are positive steps we can take if we practice the concepts of reality living.

THE WORKAHOLIC SPOUSE

When he opens the floor to questions, the marriage seminar leader always hears from at least one wife who will ask, "How do you live with a workaholic husband?" Give her a chance to explain, and she will talk about a husband who spends long hours at work and short hours at home. He leaves early in the morning and returns late at night. He sees his children only when they are asleep, and his wife sees him only when he is exhausted. He may succeed in making much money, or he may have little to show for his efforts. But his paycheck is his only contribution to the family.

I remember Andrea, whose description of her husband was almost exactly like that. By the time she had finished, numerous wives were nodding their heads, identifying with Andrea. I am not suggesting that there are not workaholic wives, but this malady afflicts males far more frequently than females.

Who is this workaholic husband? He is a man who has put all his marbles in the same bag. For him, his vocation is his life. He happens to be married and he happens, usually, to have children, but he is obsessed with his work. He doesn't understand why his wife is not happy with his accomplishments and all the material things that he provides for the family. But for the workaholic, his vocation is more than a search for daily bread—it is a search for daily meaning. His life has no balance.

Usually he enjoys his work. He bounces out of bed in the morning with an eagerness to tackle the challenges of the day. When he comes home, work fills his briefcase to keep him busy. Always busy, but seldom satisfied. Enough is never enough. The sun shines bright on another opportunity, and he must seize it before dark.

He is usually well respected in the community, and he often receives accolades from his employer. On the other hand, his wife seldom views him as Mr. Wonderful. She is likely to be critical of him because he invests so little in their relationship and is so uninvolved in the lives of the children.

CONFESSIONS OF A WORKAHOLIC

Here is the story of a self-confessed workaholic. I first met Jim in Elgin, Illinois, at one of my marriage seminars. As I often do, I asked permission to record his story. Here are excerpts of what he said.

"I was like lots of men who have the idea of making it big, of becoming somebody. I started with the idea that if I worked harder and smarter, I would get ahead. I thought that if I worked long hours and applied my mind and came up with creative ideas, I would overcome the insecurities of my youth and would get ahead of my peers. I can't say that I really liked my work, but I was good at it. In a few years I was moving up the ladder; I was reaching my goals, I was getting awards from my supervisor. But I must admit that I never felt a lot of satisfaction. I always sensed that I needed to do more.

"There were good times, of course. When I experienced the high of being salesman of the year, it felt good. I knew that everyone looked up to me. I knew that I had reached the goal that many of them were striving for. But when the euphoria of the moment was over, there was always that nagging feeling that I really should be much further ahead. When there were setbacks and I didn't do so well, I thought the only answer was to work harder.

"I spent long hours on the job, I seldom saw my kids awake. I would sneak into their bedrooms at night and look at their sleeping faces and tell myself that I was working hard to provide a good future for them. I was not there when they took their first steps nor was I there when they first rode a bicycle. My nephew had the pleasure of launching them on wheels. At the time, I didn't realize that I was missing anything. I was thrilled when I found out on Sunday that my son had ridden a bicycle that week—'without training wheels,' he said. I can hardly think about it without crying now but then, I was enthusiastic and told him how great that was. I guess in my own mind I thought he was taking the kind of steps that would one day get him where I was.

"The message I heard in my mind was 'go, go, go; work, work, work.' I didn't have time to play with my kids and seldom time to spend an evening making love to my wife. I had no friends except business acquaintances and certainly had no time for reading unless it was related to my work."

Jim noted that he did some things for his wife, like sending her a card and flowers on her birthday; but they still had little time together. Amy's complaints were frequent and made Jim want to escape even more, for "all she did was remind me of my failures as a father and husband," he said.

But one Sunday afternoon Amy got his attention with a proposed outing. She wouldn't say where they were going, only that she thought he'd like it. "It won't take long, and you don't have to change clothes. Let's go." Jim was only slightly interested but thought, *Here's an opportunity to do something she wants me to do. Maybe if I go with her, she will reciprocate with a little tenderness toward me tonight.* So Amy drove them to their destination.

As Jim explained, "She drove me to the newest, nicest retirement center I have ever seen. The lawns were absolutely beautiful; the buildings were attractive, none of the drabness one typically expects at a retirement center. We walked into the main building and saw a beautiful chandelier flanked with a baby grand piano and French provincial couches and chairs. Out back was a beautiful golf course. Amy started pointing out all of these amenities to me."

"Why did you bring me out here?" he asked. "I'm only thirty-eight; we're not about to retire anytime soon."

"But I wanted you to have a visual image of what it's going to be like, Jim, when you retire. With all the money you are making, you and I can afford to live in a place like this. We'll have a wonderful life together. You can play golf in the day and we'll make love at night. We can attend movies and symphonies. We can have a real life, Jim, and all of this in only twenty-seven more years."

"Amy," Jim said. "You are out of your mind. What are you talking about? This is absurd."

"No, I am not out of my mind, Jim. I'm very much in control of my mind and I don't intend to wait twenty-seven years to have a real life with you. By that time, the children won't know you at all and I'll be too old to have sex." Her voice was firm; her words direct: "I want you *now*, Jim, not in a retirement center. I'm tired of being a widow. I don't care if we ever live in a retirement center. I want to live now. I want us to have a life. I want the kids to be able to say, 'My dad took me fishing.'

"I don't know what you want, Jim, but if all you want is to live in this beautiful retirement center, then you'll have to live here by yourself. This is not what I want. I want a real life with you—now. I'm not asking you to quit your job; I'm asking you to find a way to live before you retire."

Amy's words stunned her husband. "I don't remember crying since I was a child, but I cried that afternoon," Jim recalled. "Standing near the eighteenth green, I cried. My life flashed before me on the screen of my mind. I heard my father telling me that I would never amount to anything. I saw the years I had invested in trying to prove him wrong, and now I realized that I was in danger of losing everything that was important to me.

"I didn't blame Amy. I knew that she was telling me the truth. And through my tears I said, 'I'm sorry. I'm sorry. I know it's all been wrong. I was doing what I thought was important. But I was wrong.'"

And Jim began what he calls "a real change in my life." For a month he analyzed what he could do about his all-consuming job. He concluded that he couldn't cut back his time there because of the pattern already in place, so he began searching for another job.

"It really was not that hard to leave when I found a new job. I've spent several years now rediscovering the real world. I've done a lot of thinking, looking back and trying to learn why I had invested so many years thinking that material success was worth paying any cost to achieve."

Jim's conclusion? "I realize now that life is relatively short and we are very foolish if we do not keep a balance between work and family. I've observed that few people are ever satisfied with their success in their vocation no matter how much they have achieved. I'm convinced we never 'make it' because the goals keep expanding ahead of you. If in trying to be a success you lose your wife and family, you've lost it all. I'll never regret the day that Amy forced me to face reality."

I must confess that by the time Jim finished his story, I had tears in my eyes, tears of joy to meet a man who had awakened from his stupor of obsessiveness with work while his wife was still there and his children still at home. I was eager to talk with Amy and find out the rest of the story. What motivated her? How did she come to her creative approach in getting Jim's attention? What had she experienced in the years before that? Later I'll tell you her side of the story, but first let's take a look at what motivates men to be workaholics. What are the inner needs that drive the people we commonly call workaholics?

FEELINGS OF INFERIORITY

Many workaholics are suffering from a deep sense of inferiority. The seeds were probably planted in childhood. The message received from parents was "You are not as good as your brother. You are not as smart as your sister. You will never make it." As a child, the son (or daughter) internalized those messages; and as an adult, the messages still play in the mind of the workaholic. His work is an effort to overcome these feelings of inferiority. If he works hard enough and well enough, he will prove to himself and others that he is not inferior. The person who overworks because he feels inferior must perform on a higher level than those around him. This often means that he must spend more hours away from home pursuing his goal of excellence.

This sense of inferiority often leads the workaholic to be a perfectionist. When he finishes a task, it seldom meets his own approval. "I just don't think my superior will be happy with this," he reasons. So he spends another hour working on an already excellent report. This perfectionist tendency is another reason why the workaholic seldom attacks problems around the house. He doesn't want to start a project because he doesn't believe that he can do it the way it ought to be done. Rather than proving himself a failure, it is better not to begin.

Many workaholics also feel unloved. The message received from parents was not "I love you," but rather "I love you if . . . . I love you if you make up your bed, put your dishes in the dishwasher, clean up your room, mow the grass, and make straight A's." Such conditional love sets a child up to become an adult workaholic.

Yes, workaholics are motivated by their need for love. And while they often receive accolades from their employers, which give them some sense of well-being, they seldom receive love from the significant people in their lives, namely their spouses and children. Unless the workaholic awakens from his obsessive behavior as did Jim, he may live a lifetime with his need for love unmet.

Another need which motivates the workaholic is the need to achieve. The workaholic is often searching for significance. He has been led to believe that the fastest way to accomplish something of lasting value is to pursue his vocation with a passion, to accumulate a successful financial portfolio, own a nice house with expensive furnishings. He is searching for significance in the wrong places, but he has not yet made that discovery.

WORKING TO AVOID CONFRONTATIONS

Some workaholics are also hiding from their spouses. They use busyness to avoid getting in touch with their own feelings or the feelings of their spouses. For some people, it is much easier to work than it is to relate to a spouse on an emotional level. Someone has said, "Men love competition but hate confrontation." Such men see confrontation with their wives as a lose/lose proposition.

A husband doesn't want his wife to lose in a confrontation because she will treat him with even greater harshness or withdrawal. He certainly doesn't want to lose the confrontation because this confirms the parental message of his incompetence. Thus, he stays at the office to avoid coming home to a wife who makes him feel incompetent as a husband or father. For the workaholic, the thought of facing a disgruntled wife is enough to keep him away until she is asleep. If he views himself as incompetent, the last thing he wants is for his wife to concur. If by virtue of his hard work he has been able to convince himself that he is a success, he certainly does not want to hear his wife rebuff him and repeat the message of his parents. If the criticism from his wife has been constant and long term, he may have concluded that he will never please her; thus, he invests his energy in his vocation where he has some measure of success and recognition.

Of course, working wives can become workaholics, too. Often they stay at work, either at the office or in the home study, in order to hide from their husbands and avoid a confrontation. Some women also become workaholics to escape a spouse's condemnation; they choose to work long hours away from their husbands.

When it comes to working to avoid condemnation, even religious service can become an escape. Ministers often fall into this category. Their obsession becomes serving God. Their view of God as a holy creature who demands perfection or at least demands that their good deeds outweigh the bad deeds keeps them diligently working to please God. Ironically, this is the opposite of the true Christian message; yet many ministers and parishioners read the Bible through the grid of parental condemnation and perfectionistic expectations. Thus, they work hard in the service of God.

One minister's wife said to me, "My husband preaches against adultery but in fact, he is committing adultery. I don't mean he is having an affair with a woman; I mean the church has become his mistress. I am his housekeeper and our children are orphans. Everyone praises him for being such a wonderful pastor. He is 'always available.' I'm sorry, but I don't share the view of the congregation. I can't believe that it pleases God for him to give his family so little attention while he ministers to others."

I listened, and helped the wife decide on action that would catch the ears and heart of her husband. The answer came as this minister joined 50,000 other men at a football stadium for a Promise Keepers conference. Promise Keepers is a national men's movement, which has a strong emphasis upon the husband's responsibility in the home. The husband listened as an African American football player talked about the importance of the male's role in the Afro-American family. As a bolt of lightning, the pastor's heart was struck with his failure in his own family. He had heard the voice of God. Later when the speaker asked that the men turn to another man and "confess their faults one to another," the lady's husband turned to his fellow pastor and confessed that he had failed his wife and children. That was the beginning of a radical change in his ministry—and their marriage.

AMY'S COMPLAINTS

Of course, the workaholic is a very responsible person; that may even be part of the initial attraction to his or her mate. For instance, Amy described her earlier years with Jim, before their dramatic confrontation on the lawn of the retirement center.

"Jim was twenty-four when we got married," she said, "and I was twenty-three. I was so in love with him. He was my ideal of a hardworking man. He had accomplished much since finishing college, and I knew that we would have a wonderful life together. During courtship, he was everything I had dreamed of—kind, courteous, thoughtful, attentive, and yes, good-looking. I knew he would be a perfect husband.

"The first two years of our marriage were exciting. We were buying a house, getting the furniture, getting settled in. But then, Jim got a promotion. From that point on, it seemed like everything changed. We had more money but saw less of each other."

Amy didn't like what was happening with his time, and she told Jim that. "I felt like the job was more important than I was. He assured me that it wouldn't be like this forever but that the next two or three years were going to require a lot of his time. I understood that and I was willing to sacrifice if it were temporary.

"In a year or so, the baby came and my life was absorbed with caring for the baby. Jim's mother and my mother gave me a lot of help the first year. Actually, I think their help maintained my stability. They often baby-sat while I got away for some relaxation. I even met Jim for lunch a few times. Those were special times. But then Jim's parents moved out of town and my mother got sick. I really needed Jim but he was not there for me. Three years had passed but things were worse than ever."

When she began to complain once more, Jim said that she didn't appreciate his hard work. "You should be thankful for all that I provide for you and the baby," he told her.

"I was thankful but I didn't feel that we were living a normal life," Amy told me. "I felt that Jim was obsessed with his work and that I certainly was not at the top of his list of priorities."

Her husband, whose hardworking approach had first attracted her, seemed to be moving out of control. For the next several years, Amy responded by alternating between an aggressive and passive approach. "Part of the time, I would give him angry lectures, accuse him of not loving me, even accused him once of having an affair. I told him that he would live to regret the day he got that job. I complained about the job, I criticized his superiors, I told him about my lack of respect for the administration of a company that would require a man to spend so much time at work. Then I would go for long periods of time saying nothing, but suffering and showing by my behavior that I was unhappy with Jim and our relationship. During these times, we had fewer arguments, but the pain was more intense for me. I steadily grew to a place of hopelessness. I really had come to believe that Jim really didn't care."

A LOVING SOLUTION FOR AMY AND JIM

Change came when she read a book about inner motives behind people's behavior. She began to realize, as she put it, "Jim's behavior had little to do with me and far more to do with him. I remembered the stories he told me when we were dating, of how his father criticized his school work and his athletic efforts. I remembered specific stories about his father such as the Saturday Jim washed the car and his father came out and pointed out a spot he had missed.

"His father was seldom complimentary and almost always critical. There was no question about it; Jim had gotten the message as a child that he was not good enough and that his father was not pleased with him.

"For the first time, I realized that much of Jim's motivation for working so much was to prove to his father that he 'could make it.' He was trying to prove his own self-worth and I realized that his plan was working. The accomplishments he made on the job were giving him the affirmation he needed from others, and I really believed that Jim was feeling good about his accomplishments. The problem, of course, was that I was feeling left out."

Amy also realized that her critical attitude was much like that of Jim's father's and that she was driving Jim away by her critical comments about his work. So she decided to stop making critical comments and start giving Jim positive comments about his job.

"I started telling him the good things I heard people say about his company. I started saying things like, 'Your supervisor must be very proud of you. You must have saved the company thousands of dollars with that decision.' I started expressing appreciation for the way he provided for me and the children. I started giving him the affirmation which I knew he needed.

"Over a period of a couple of months, the atmosphere between the two of us began to improve. We weren't having fights and Jim seemed to enjoy the few times we went out to dinner. But his work patterns did not change. I felt that I had changed my attitude and I had stopped my negative behavior and had started giving positive affirmation. But it didn't seem to be influencing Jim to make any changes."

So what made Amy think of the visit to the retirement center? A friend of hers suggested Amy try using "tough love," saying that love sometimes must be hard and firm and that if we really care about someone, we will confront the person in a kind but firm way. "I thought about it for a long time and I realized that Jim was a good man but that unless he was shocked, his obsession with work was not going to change.

"So I thought about a creative way that I could break the news to him that I was very unhappy with our relationship and unwilling to continue in the present mode. I felt that over the past couple of months, I had demonstrated my soft love for him by changing my behavior. Now it was time for tough love.

"What I said to him at the retirement center was a speech I had rehearsed many times. I said it with emotion, I said it with sincerity, and I said it with firmness. Thank God, he listened."

Later Jim agreed to go with Amy for marriage counseling. And the counselor helped Jim in making the decision to find another vocation that would be less time demanding and would give him the freedom to start over with a more balanced perspective on life. Amy calls that and other changes by Jim "pretty radical," but very helpful to their marriage.

With a twinkle in her eye, Amy told me, "I am actually looking forward to living with him at the retirement center. I'm just glad I don't have to wait till then to start living."

Jim said, "I'm not sure we can afford to live at that retirement center. It doesn't matter. Wherever we are, we are going to enjoy our relationship."

I want to conclude this chapter by saying that I believe that Amy's efforts at soft and tender love were important before she came to her tough love approach. Jim may not have had the same response on the eighteenth green of the retirement center golf course if Amy had not recognized Jim's inner need for significance and self-worth, understood the role of his father's condemning messages in motivating him to become a workaholic, and stopped her critical remarks about his work, replacing them with affirming words. I believe that tough love must always be preceded by tender love.

Remember, love is looking out for the other person's interest. The first step is trying to understand the behavior of your spouse, the inner motivations that drive him or her, and then asking yourself whether your past responses to that negative behavior have actually made the problem worse. Most of the time, the first step in becoming a positive change agent in a troubled marriage is to change our own attitude based on a better understanding of our spouse's behavior. When we change our thinking and our negative responses, we become free to take a new approach. These new approaches, based on reality living, hold the greatest potential for influencing your spouse to make positive changes.

THE CONTROLLING SPOUSE

$\mathcal{A}$n overly controlling spouse is the source of many troubled marriages. Remember Jodie in chapter 1? A classmate of mine in high school, Jodie visited with me more than thirty years later during one of my marriage seminars near St. Louis. She recounted the pain of her twenty-seven-year marriage to Roger, a hardworking man who had been successful in his vocation but a failure in his marriage. Jodie had dreamed of a partnership where she and Roger could share thoughts, feelings, desires, and work together as a team in facing life. Roger, on the other hand, was an obsessive controller. He had no concept of teamwork. His father was extremely domineering and he was repeating the model of his father.

Listen to Jodie's words again. "He controls the money like he is a guard at Fort Knox. I have to ask for every nickel. Every time I come home he wants to know where I've been and what I've done. . . . He has to have the final decision in everything. Our social life is almost nil because he never wants to do anything with anyone else. He's told our children that he will not pay for their college unless they go to the university of his choice. Gary, I feel like I am a bird in a cage. Actually, I feel like a hamster in a cage—I don't have wings anymore."

In further conversation, I found out that Jodie had been suffering from anxiety attacks for the past two or three years. She described these attacks in the following way. "I get short of breath and my chest gets tight. I feel like I am suffocating. They come on with no warning and render me helpless." The anxiety attacks had led her to seek counseling. The counselor was suggesting that the attacks might be directly related to the stress under which she was living in her marriage. Jodie didn't want to admit it, but she knew the counselor was correct. The emotional stress under which she had lived for many years was now expressing itself in physical symptoms. The counselor referred her to a medical doctor for medication, but she and the counselor knew that this was not the long-term answer to her problem. Something had to change in her troubled marriage.

A MODEL FROM CHILDHOOD

Following a Parental Model

Who are these controlling men (and sometimes women) who seek to dominate their spouses? Many times they are some of the most respected people in the community, and often they are unaware of their controlling behavior. They are simply following a lifestyle which to them seems normal. They are either living out the model that they observed in childhood or they are following the script written in their personality. Let's look at each of these.

Roger, Jodie's husband, fell into the first category. His father was an authoritarian role model. He made the money and he ran the house. The only decisions his wife made were how to dress the kids and what the family would eat. Even in these areas, he sometimes criticized her. All other decisions Roger's father made himself. He prided himself on being a successful man and ruling his family well. His children were respected in the community and his wife was viewed as a lovely lady. The whole family was active in the local church, and Roger's dad often related his controlling behavior to the biblical mandate that "the husband is the head of the wife." His father exuded self-confidence and was known as a man who made things happen.

Roger's mother in the early days had complained about his controlling behavior, but that was before Roger was born. After the children came, she busied herself with the children and accepted her lot in life. She was pleased that her husband was a good provider, and she never questioned any of his decisions. If she disagreed, she kept her thoughts to herself, and in due time her pained emotions would subside. She did not have an intimate emotional relationship with Roger's dad, but she assumed that her marriage was pretty much like that of all the ladies she knew.

Roger was simply following the model with which he had grown up. He was a hard worker and a good provider, so he wondered why Jodie was complaining. Why was she not willing to play her role as well as he was playing his? He reasoned that, while in college, she had picked up feminist ideas, although he never expressed that thought to Jodie.

If you had confronted Roger, he would never have admitted that his behavior was controlling. He was simply doing what a man does. He could not have understood why Jodie would have felt anything but gratitude. Why shouldn't she be grateful? She could not ask for a better husband than he. Unfortunately, Roger never changed his mind. Two years later, I got a note from Jodie telling me that she and Roger were divorced and that she had married a "wonderful" man.

THE DOMINATING PERSONALITY

There is another kind of individual who is not likely to recognize his/her controlling patterns. This is the person who has what psychologists often call a dominating or controlling personality. This person is not following the model of parents; he is playing out the script that is written in his personality.

These are people who often become leaders in the community, on the job, or in the church. They are the kind of people who take authority, solve problems, make decisions, and get things done. They are movers and shakers. Usually they have a high level of self-confidence and believe they can accomplish anything. Give them a task and it will be done. They produce results. However, dominating persons are not in touch with emotions—their own or others'. Their attitude is, "What difference does it make how you feel? Let's get on with the job."

If someone disagrees with a dominating personality, that person is seen as an obstacle in reaching the goal. The dominant personality is always ready to argue and convince the opponent that he is wrong. If the dominant person cannot convince the opponent, he or she will sometimes intimidate him—whatever is necessary to reach the goal. Dominant personalities are goal-oriented, not relationship-oriented. They get things done, but they often hurt people in the process. To them, that is simply part of the cost of reaching the objective.

They are often rigid in their orientation. Their attitude is "There is only one thing to do—finish the task. There is only one way to do it—my way; and there is only one time to do it—now." They are often driven by a sense of obligation or duty. Once they have accepted a task, they do not want to be bothered with such questions as "Why are we doing this?" And once they have a plan in action, they don't want to be slowed with questions such as "Is this the best way to do it?" Get the Job Done and As Efficiently As Possible is their motto. These people accomplish much in the corporation and community.

When the person with a dominating personality marries, he or she brings that personality into the marriage and does what comes naturally. Getting married itself was a task for this individual. Before the wedding, the dominating personality did whatever was necessary to reach the goal; after the wedding, the task was accomplished. Now it is time for another task. Thus, there is often drastic behavior change in this person after marriage. Many wives testify that once the wedding day was past, the man they married was gone forever.

In the marriage, the dominating personality will make decisions quickly, often not involving the spouse in the decision at all. "Why bother him? I can get this done. Let him spend his energies somewhere else" is the attitude. If the spouse confronts the dominating partner about not being involved in the decisions, the partner is amazed it is an issue. "It's something I could handle. Why would you want to waste your time talking about it?" In the dominating person's mind, he is not controlling but being efficient.

PHILLIP, THE EFFICIENCY EXPERT

Phillip was this kind of husband. Early in life, he decided that he wanted to retire at fifty. He was an engineer with a good job, on a fast track toward promotion. He felt good about his accomplishments on the job, and he also applied his skills in managing finances at home. He put himself and his wife on a strict budget. In his mind, he was allowing plenty for food, clothing, maintenance, etc. He included a monthly amount for recreation and even some "spending money" for himself and his wife. He covered all the bases and the budget was extremely efficient.

The problem was Sally did not agree with the budget. Phillip saw her objections as a threat to his leadership and an affront to his skills. He was willing to explain the budget to her one time but when she still did not agree, he became angry and withdrew. He knew his plan was workable; why was she making such a fuss? Eventually, Sally stopped talking about it, and he took her silence as acquiescence. So he moved on to apply his efficient planning to other areas of money management.

He analyzed the household to determine how to get the most efficiency out of all appliances. He put water-saver shower heads on all the showers. He made improvements on the windows in order to get the best rate from the electric company. He installed efficiency filters on the furnace. Later, he got a wood stove, which in his mind would save a large amount on heating cost. That was when Sally exploded again. But eventually his arguments and logic quieted her opposition, and he moved on to the next task.

Once the house was efficient, he applied his skills to the world of investment. He began to make investments that he believed to be safe but also held the potential for huge gains. Again Sally disagreed, but by now she knew she had no chance of succeeding with Phillip. She voiced her opinion but withdrew in silence.

Phillip had now covered the key areas: a good job making

good money, the household running efficiently, and making good investments. He was well on the way to his goal of retirement at fifty. He would not have admitted he was a controller; he was simply doing what to him was perfectly natural.

Phillip's neat world was shattered the evening he came home and found Sally's clothes and much of the furniture moved out of the house and this note lying on the kitchen table:

Dear Phillip,

I would like to be able to say I love you very much, but I'm not really sure what my feelings are at this point. We have been married for twenty-one years, and in the beginning we had some good years. But as time went on, I felt that you became more and more controlling. In recent years, I have felt that I am not a part of your life. You never ask my advice and if I give it, you always tell me why I am wrong. You've got the house running so efficiently and saving so much money that I can hardly get the soap off my back when I take a shower, the water is so weak. The wooden stove keeps me coughing constantly. I have decided that you can have your efficient house. I've got me an apartment with plenty of water and fresh air.

I know you see yourself as a good provider and a solid husband. You probably wonder why I would do what I am doing. I guess that goes to show that you really haven't heard me through all these years. I have pleaded with you to let me be a part of your life, to treat me as an individual, to let my ideas count for something, but it has become obvious that the only ideas that matter in our marriage are your ideas. My feelings and my thoughts are unimportant. I thought for a long time that you were probably right—that I didn't have any good thoughts or good feelings. I know now that you are wrong. Everybody deserves the right to think and feel and if they are married, to express those thoughts and feelings to their spouse and to be respected. I feel no respect from you. I feel that you have treated me as a child for many years. I'm tired of being a child; I want to be an adult. I know that I will never be an adult with you. Therefore, I'm leaving.

Don't expect me to come back. I've thought about this for a long time. I know that you will never change. Maybe you cannot change. I know that I cannot spend the rest of my life living with you. I hope you can retire at fifty, and I hope you find somebody who will enjoy your controlling personality. But that someone cannot be me.

The letter was signed simply "Sally." Phillip read the letter ten times that night. He was incredulous. He could not believe what he was reading. *What is she talking about—"controlling behavior"?* he wondered. *I have done all of this for us.* Indeed he had envisioned them having a wonderful life together after he retired. He thought they were having a wonderful life now. *Why is she criticizing my efforts to be efficient? What is she talking about—treating her like a child? What does she mean—I didn't listen to her? I did listen, but I'm not going to do what she wants if I know it's not the best thing to do.*

Phillip knew there was no need to try to find Sally that night. He knew that he and she needed time to think about what she had done. He decided that he would get a good night's sleep and tomorrow, he would decide his strategy. Not surprisingly, he slept rather well that night. He knew in his mind that he would come up with a plan, and if he could just talk to Sally, he could help her understand that she was wrong and needed to come home.

The next day, he spent much of his time trying to figure how he could find Sally and talk to her.

On his lunch hour he took his first step in his search-and-find strategy. He called Sally's best friend, knowing that she would know where Sally was. But the friend refused to tell him, so Phillip quickly shifted to Plan B. He told Sally's friend how deeply hurt he was and how he could not believe what Sally had done. He emphasized how much he needed to talk to Sally and asked the friend to ask her if she would call him. The friend agreed, and Phillip felt that his first step had been somewhat successful.

However, when Sally did not call that night, he became more anxious. But not wanting to appear panicky, he decided not to call her friend but to watch football on television. He reasoned that if she didn't call tonight, he would call another friend tomorrow. His efforts to search and find went on for a week, but he was not successful in locating Sally.

The next week, he received legal separation papers delivered to him by the local sheriff's department. Again, he sat at the kitchen table reading a document from Sally, this one far more formal, impersonal, and unemotional. Again, his response was "This is unbelievable. I cannot believe she is doing this." He said the words out loud and then said to himself, *Doesn't she realize what she is doing? All I have worked for through the years will be destroyed. She is throwing it all away and we are so close to our goal. How could she do this? She must be involved with someone else.* This thought had never crossed his mind before but the more he thought about it, the more it seemed the only logical explanation for Sally's behavior. Again, he called Sally's best friend, told her about the separation papers and openly asked her, "Is Sally having an affair? It's the only reason I can think of that she would do something like this."

"Phillip, I can assure you Sally is not having an affair," Sally's friend answered. "I think if you will read her letter again you will understand why she is doing this. I think she has felt so controlled for so long that she found it emotionally unbearable. I don't know if she is right or not, but I do know that this is what she is feeling."

"I don't understand that," Phillip said. "Everything I have ever done has always been for her benefit." The friend responded, "I guess that is not the way she sees it, Phillip." The next day Phillip decided he would get a lawyer. *If this is what she wants, then I have got to protect myself. Otherwise, she will take everything I've got.*

So the legal battle began between two lawyers. The motivating force was Phillip's efforts to reach his goal of retiring. He would not make it by fifty but maybe when all this was over, he would make it by fifty-five. Over the next month, Phillip kept himself busy with work, keeping the house in order, and going to church meetings. He wanted everyone to know that this separation was not his idea, that he couldn't understand what had gotten into Sally.

Six weeks after Sally left, Phillip had still not seen Sally nor heard from her. Then one night, it happened in the most unlikely place. He was at the local Wal-Mart when he looked up and there was Sally. She saw him at the same time he saw her. He started walking toward her slowly and when he was close enough he said, "Hi," and Sally responded, "Hi." They looked at each other in silence for what seemed like an eternity and then Phillip said, "Sally, I don't understand all of this. I don't know why you have chosen to do all of this but I do know that I still love you. Could we get together and talk?" To his surprise, Sally agreed.

On Friday night, they met for a meal. During the meal, they shared with each other how things were going on their jobs. After eating, Phillip gave Sally a lecture on how illogical all of this was, on how they were going to lose everything he had worked for through all the years. He told her how devastating this was to the children (all of whom were now grown). He reminded her that this was not the Christian thing to do and expressed his concern about her faith in God.

A Life Being Crushed

When he finished his lecture, Sally did not respond to any of his arguments. Rather she said to him what she had wanted to say for many years. She poured out her pain of what it was like to live under his dominating influence. She told him that her life was being crushed out of her by his controlling behavior. She gave numerous examples—all the pain, the hurt, the frustration came back to her and she was able to verbalize it to Phillip. When she finished, Phillip was silent for a long time and then he started shaking his head and said softly and slowly, "I never knew you felt that way," to which Sally responded, "I told you many times, Phillip. I told you *many* times."

"I guess I never really heard you," said Phillip. By this time, Sally said, "I think I need to go now." As they stood on the sidewalk in front of the restaurant, Phillip said, "Sally, can't we work this out? I can change. Why don't you come home and let's work on it?"

"For many years, I hoped you would change but you never did. It got worse instead of better. I cannot live with you. It's not easy for you to change. If it were, you would have changed years ago."

Phillip didn't press the issue but he did tell her that he appreciated her seeing him tonight and it was good to talk with her. They went to their separate cars and drove away in opposite directions.

Following this initial contact, Sally and Phillip had several dinners together over the next few months, Phillip always pleading that she drop the separation and move home; Sally insisting that there was no hope. Finally one night she said, "Phillip, if you are really serious, then I am going to suggest that you get counseling from someone who understands how to work with people who have controlling personalities, because even after all of our talks, I don't think you understand what I am saying. I'm not promising you that I will come back if you will get counseling; I am saying that I will never come back unless you get counseling."

Two weeks later, Phillip had an appointment with a counselor and began an extended process of self-discovery. He had never read books on psychology or relationships. But in a few weeks, he was discovering things about himself that he had never known, and he was beginning to understand why Sally had felt so controlled and oppressed. In due time, he was not only apologizing to his wife, but he was sharing with her his insights about himself, and he was acknowledging that now he finally understood why she had taken the steps she had taken. He realized how oppressive his behavior had become. He told her that he would never try to force her to come back but that he would like to ask that they do some marriage counseling and see if there were any possibility of rebuilding their marriage.

After two weeks of thought, prayer, and talking with her own counselor, Sally agreed to begin marriage counseling. Seven months later, she and Phillip reaffirmed their vows to each other and she moved back home. She had no sense that she was capitulating nor did she have the sense that she had won a victory over him. She did have a deep confidence that, together, they had discovered not only the problems in their troubled marriage but also answers. Both of them had grown tremendously through the process, and she had every confidence that life together would be different in the future.

All of this happened ten years ago, and Phillip and Sally now agree that it has been the happiest ten years of their lives. Neither of them are anticipating retirement. They are seeking to make the most of each day in their mutually supportive marriage.

Did Phillip lose his dominating personality? The answer is no, but he now understands it and understands that he must control his natural desires to dominate. He is also sensitive to how his actions affect others, especially Sally. It is not his desire to control her. Sally now has the freedom to share her emotions with him and if some statement or action on his part stimulates a sense of control within her, she can share this with Phillip without fear of his response. She can predict that he will say, "Tell me about it. I want to understand what you are thinking and feeling." They are discovering how fulfilling a relationship can be when two people learn to respect each other, acknowledge differences, have genuine concern for the feelings and thoughts of the other, and seek to work together as a team for the mutual benefit of both.

THE CHOICE TO LEAVE

Let me make two important observations about Sally's actions. Before taking the step to leave Phillip, she had been in counseling for four months. She had shared with the counselor all the pain, frustration, and ambivalent feelings she experienced through the years. She had begun to build her own self-confidence and sense of significance, which had been beaten down by Phillip's controlling behavior through the years. She was now emotionally strong enough to apply the principles of reality living. She took responsibility for her own attitude and realized that the way she thought would influence her actions. She knew that she could not change Phillip but she could influence him. All of her efforts at talking to him had been futile. She did not know that he would respond positively to her leaving, but she knew that she had to make that effort.

She understood that her actions were not controlled by her emotions. Her strongest emotion was fear. *How will this affect the children? What will people think? Can I make it financially?* If she had listened to her emotions she would not have taken the hard step of tough love, but she knew that she was not controlled by her emotions. She also acknowledged that she had not been a perfect wife and knew that her own imperfections did not mean that she was a failure or that her troubled marriage was her fault. Leaving Phillip was the most loving thing she knew to do. She prayed that the results would be positive. Most spouses who have lived with a highly controlling person for a long period of time will need the guidance of a counselor to take the kind of steps that Sally took.

The second observation is that a highly controlling person who has dominated a spouse for many years does not change quickly. Even after Sally left, Phillip's early efforts were at manipulating her into coming home. At this point, he had almost no understanding of the problem. He was simply playing out the script of his personality: "If there is a problem, let's fix it." Sally did not yield to this pressure and gave him no hope of coming back. She had no assurance that Phillip would eventually understand and deal with his problem, but she knew that she could not settle for anything less than radical healing of the relationship.

Are there actions less radical than separation that hold the potential for influencing a controlling spouse to make positive changes? The answer is yes, and those actions should always be tried fully before taking the tough love approach that Sally took. But first, let's look at two common negative approaches which people take to a controlling spouse.

TWO NEGATIVE WAYS TO HANDLE A CONTROLLING SPOUSE

The first negative approach is the power play. The attitude is "two people can play this game." If you are going to try to control me, I will fight you to the end. This approach leads to angry, heated arguments in which you try to out-argue the controlling spouse. The more the controller argues, the more you argue. No one ever wins, but the power play goes on. When the argument is over, you try to stay as uninvolved as possible over the next few days. Eventually there is another power play and the arguing continues. Many couples have followed this pattern for years; it obviously perpetuates a troubled marriage.

The second negative approach is what I call the submissive-servant approach. The attitude is "I yield to the controller and avoid conflict." The motto is "Peace at Any Price." This essentially renders the person a slave to the controller's demands. Ironically, the submissive-servant approach does not make for peace. It simply plays out the battle inside the spouse who is being controlled. Externally the couple seems to be at peace but nothing could be further from the truth. This also perpetuates a troubled marriage.

THE POSITIVE WAY TO RESPOND TO A CONTROLLING SPOUSE

However, there is a healthy approach based upon understanding the needs of the controlling personality and your own needs. First, understand that the highly controlling person is one who has taken the need for freedom too far. The need for freedom is legitimate but when one is concerned only for his own freedom with no concern for how it may take away from the freedom of another, he has become an abusive controller. Any positive solution to influencing the controller must deal with his/her freedom, but it must also provide freedom for the spouse.

Second, understand and respond to the controller's need for significance. The self-worth of most controllers is tied to their performance. The more often they reach the tasks and goals they have set, the better they feel about themselves. For the controller, failure to reach the goal is interpreted as "I am a failure." Thus, the inner needs for freedom and significance must be addressed by the spouse who would seek to be a change agent in influencing the controller.

Let me suggest an approach that has proven successful for many. You do not influence a controller by argument. Argument to a controller is like throwing gasoline on a fire. The controller is already strongly motivated to reach his/her goal. Your argument is simply one more obstacle in reaching that goal. It fires his engine to overcome your argument and prove that his way is the best way. You will not argue long enough or well enough to influence a controller. The approach I have found most helpful is what I call *influencing by agreement*. You agree with the controller's arguments but you don't allow yourself to be controlled by those arguments.

I hear someone objecting, "Agree with their arguments? I can't possibly do that." The reality is you can almost always agree with the arguments of your spouse. Why? Because their arguments are correct, from their perspective. For example, all of Phillip's energy-conserving, money-saving ideas were correct from one perspective, namely, saving money. Therefore, the *influence by agreement approach* would lead Sally to say something like this, "Phillip, I really appreciate your efforts to save money. I think your goal to retire at fifty is a worthy goal. I'm sure that it will save some money to use the water-saver shower heads; but I cannot afford to take thirty minutes to get the shampoo out of my hair. I want to help you save money and if you will figure how much money we are saving by using the 'water-saver' shower heads, I'll be happy to take that amount out of the food budget each month. From the money-saving perspective, it is a great idea, but from the practical perspective it makes life really difficult for me."

If Phillip persists with other arguments, she agrees with all of his arguments but insists that it is not a comfort which she is willing to sacrifice. If Phillip hasn't changed the shower head in a week, she calls a plumber and has the old head reinstalled. Chances are Phillip will mumble about how she's wasting money, but he will not reinstall the water-saving shower head.

Influencing by agreement and yet not allowing oneself to be controlled holds tremendous potential for influencing a controlling spouse. First, this approach does not strike at the self-worth or significance of the controller. It is not arguing that his ideas are bad, which he will always interpret as personal criticism and will fight to prove that his ideas are worthy. Influencing by agreement virtually eliminates arguing rather than fueling its fire. It actually builds up the spouse's self-esteem because it affirms his purposes and agrees with his ideas.

However, it is extremely important to follow through with the second half of this approach and not allow oneself to be controlled by the controller. When you assert your own freedom to make decisions, you are helping your spouse understand by your actions that freedom is a two-way street and that all of us need a measure of freedom. You are not demanding total freedom nor are you yielding such freedom to the controller. Once the controller sees that you have a mind of your own and you will not be controlled by his or her limited perspective, your mate will likely come to respect your freedom. This approach applied consistently over a period of time has influenced many controllers to a more balanced approach to life.

Another approach that offers promise in positively influencing a controlling spouse is to *play to his or her strengths*. In the world of sports and business, good coaches and supervisors always follow this principle. The idea is to find the strengths of the player or employee and utilize these to the maximum. The principle also works in marriage and is especially helpful in influencing the controller. Since she is performance-oriented, she responds well to challenges to reach a given goal. Therefore, a controlling spouse will welcome a request for help. "I have observed that you are really good at mapping out strategies to reach goals. Would you be willing to help me with a project? A friend of mind has asked me to come up with practical ideas on how she and her husband can enrich their marriage. I have some ideas, but would you give some thought to that and next week, pool our ideas?"

You may be surprised at the ideas the controller will produce. Ideas often include: reading and discussing a book on marriage, attending a marriage enrichment seminar, setting aside a time each day for conversation, having a date night once a week with each other, buying your spouse a gift even when there is no special occasion, taking walks together, expressing appreciation to each other, etc. Once the list is made and you pass it on to your friend, you may begin trying to initiate some of these in your own marriage. Having been a part of the idea, the controller is far more likely to be willing to pursue such activities.

Because controllers are task-oriented, they are often willing to read books or attend seminars because they see this as a means of gaining information. If they can be influenced to turn their natural skills toward improving the marriage, you may be the benefactor as well as they. However, one of the tendencies of the controller when he or she thinks of marriage enrichment is to think in terms of changes the spouse needs to make. You may feel his controlling power even in these efforts. When this happens, it is time to use the *influence by agreement* approach discussed above. You agree with his ideas but you don't allow him to treat you as a slave.

In summary, arguing and fighting with a controlling spouse is the worst possible approach. You can never win an argument with a controller; you only prolong the battle. Influencing by agreement and playing to his or her strengths are much more positive approaches. Both assume a kind but firm refusal to be controlled. Individuals who would be positive change agents with a controlling spouse must accept responsibility for their own attitudes. Remember, you cannot change your spouse but you can influence him or her.

CHAPTER NINE

THE UNCOMMUNICATIVE SPOUSE

*J*ill was a free-spirited, laughing, loving, and caring person. In her office, the other secretaries tried to take their break when Jill was on break because they enjoyed her positive spirit. But in my office, Jill was not laughing. Tears long held inside were now cascading down her normally cheerful face. "Mike won't talk to me," she said. "I mean, he really won't talk to me," she sobbed. "It's tearing me up inside.

"I'm usually a happy person," she continued. "I can adapt and get along with almost anyone, but I don't know what to do when Mike won't talk to me. I ask him 'What's wrong?' and he sits there in silence as though I said nothing. Last night I told him, 'Mike, we have got to talk. We cannot go on like this.' He got up and left the room."

"How long has this been going on?" I inquired.

"It started last Sunday night when I told him that I wanted to spend the weekend at the beach with two of the girls I work with. One of the girls' parents owns a place at the beach; it wouldn't cost us anything. It would be a good chance for us to spend some time together and relax. Mike went ballistic. He told me that as a married woman, I had no right going to the beach with girls. He said that if I were going to the beach, we needed to go together. He said, 'Why would you even want to go to the beach with girls from work? Is there something going on that I don't know about?'

"Dr. Chapman, I've never been unfaithful to Mike. I don't even have such a thought. Why does he accuse me of that? I told him he was being immature and that he had no right to tell me that I couldn't go to the beach. After all, he spends most Saturdays hunting with his friend.

"We're not leaving until Friday after work, and I'll be home Sunday night. He will hardly even miss me. We went to bed angry that night and since then, Mike has not said a word to me. That was a week ago last night."

"Has Mike ever been silent like this before?" I asked.

"Two or three times," she said, "but usually just for a day or maybe two. Never this long."

"Does he talk when you are not having conflicts like this?" I asked.

"Well, he doesn't talk as much as I do," Jill said. "He's rather quiet, but he does talk. I don't have any complaints normally. But his silence is driving me crazy."

"What are you feeling toward Mike right now?" I asked.

"I don't understand him," she said. "I feel that he is trying to control my life. I don't know why he would do that. I don't try to control him. Last fall, he went fishing for a week with his friends at the beach. I didn't get bent out of shape. That was fine with me. I think he needs some time with his friends, but I need time with my friends also. Why would he get so upset about my going to the beach with my friends? And why will he not talk with me?"

"Do you think Mike would come to see me and talk about this?" I asked.

"I don't think so, Dr. Chapman. He thinks that talking to other people about your problems is a sign of weakness. He has always said that he can solve his own problems."

"Does Mike know that you came to see me today?" I asked.

"No, and if he did he would be horrified," she said.

HER NEEDS, HIS NEEDS

Jill and Mike had only been married about a year. They had attended the marriage preparation classes that I had taught, so I knew a little bit about Mike's personality. So I said to Jill, "It may be necessary later on for me to talk to Mike but let's try something first. Much of our behavior in marriage is motivated by unmet emotional needs. For example, you came to my office today because of unmet needs in your own life. You want to have an intimate, open, caring, loving relationship with Mike and right now, you don't have that. All of us need to feel loved but at the moment, you don't feel that Mike is loving you. Rather, you feel that he is trying to control your behavior.

"Another need which all of us have is the need for freedom. Mike's efforts to keep you from going to the beach are removing your sense of freedom; thus, two of your deepest emotional needs are not being met—the need for freedom and the need for love."

I explained that with those two needs unmet, she probably felt hurt, anger, disappointment, frustration, and maybe several other emotions. "Your response was to talk to me about the problem and seek a resolution." I asked her, "Does all of this make sense to you?"

"Yes, I think I understand what you're saying," she said.

"Now, Mike is also a person who has emotional needs. His behavior can also be explained in terms of unmet needs. He has the need to be loved by you, to feel that he is number one in your life. My guess is that he does not feel that at the moment. He may feel that the ladies with whom you are going to the beach are more important to you than he, that you love them more than you love him. Thus, one of his fundamental emotional needs is unmet at the moment—the need for love."

I suggested his silent treatment was his way of telling her, "This is a serious problem." His silence could also be an effort to manipulate her into agreeing not to go to the beach. "He may have used this approach with his parents during his childhood or teenage years," I said. "Perhaps his parents have caved into his desires when he gave them the silent treatment."

"I saw that twice when we were dating," Jill replied. "His mother didn't like his silence, and she ended up doing what he wanted."

"Then maybe we've discovered a learned behavior pattern in Mike's life that needs to be changed. The ideal," I said, "is to find a way where you can meet Mike's need for emotional love and at the same time maintain your own freedom. In a healthy marriage, spouses learn to meet each other's emotional needs. To the degree that this is done, a marriage is healthy. What I want and I think what you want is a healthy marriage." Jill nodded.

Then I asked her if she knew Mike's primary love language. We had discussed the five love languages during the premarital classes, and Jill felt confident it was physical touch. So I asked her to think back over the last month. "Now I want you to answer this question: 'How effective have I been in speaking Mike's primary love language over the past four weeks?'"

Jill thought for a moment and said, "Dr. Chapman, we've been so busy that I have to admit that I've not spoken his language very much in the last month. I hadn't really thought about it, but I can see now what you're talking about. Mike's love tank is probably sitting on empty. Therefore, he is threatened by my going to the beach. He feels unloved and like I'm deserting him." (That's the moment of insight that counselors wait for, when people see their situation clearly and understand what needs to be done.)

LOVING SOLUTIONS

Then I suggested the following: "What if you go home and say to Mike something like this: 'Mike, I want you to know that I love you very much. I have been thinking about us a lot since our argument on Sunday night, and I have realized that I have not spoken your primary love language very well in the last few weeks. It's not because I don't want to; it's because I've been so busy I just haven't taken time to be with you and express my love to you. I think that your opposition to my going to the beach is largely because I have not filled your love tank. I thought at first that you were trying to control my life but I really don't believe that's true.

"'I know that I give you freedom to go fishing with your friends, and I believe that you want to give me freedom to be with my friends. I also want you to know that your silence this week and unwillingness to talk with me has caused me great pain and hurt because it communicates to me that you don't love me. I feel like you have treated me as a nonhuman, and I want you to know that I find your silence very distasteful. I'm going to request that you never do this again because it hurts me so deeply, and I can tell you that I will never let you control my behavior by such silence.

"'I am going to the beach next month with my friends, but we have three weeks before that weekend. I want to show you my love. I want to hold you and kiss you and hug you and be sexually intimate with you. Hey, we can have sex every day between now and then if you desire. (Jill caught my humor and she was smiling now.) Mike, I love you, and I'm so sorry that we wasted this week in our lives. Now, how about a kiss and a hug for starters?'

"If Mike doesn't respond to this approach, then I want you to tell him that you are going to call me and come in for an appointment, that you are not going on with the silent treatment. Once you've called me and set the appointment, you invite him to come with you. If he won't come, you come alone. Now he has the knowledge that you've seen me and the next day, I will call him and ask him to come in and talk with me about the situation. I think he will come because I think Mike respects me." She nodded.

"I think he'd come, Dr. Chapman, but I want to try the other approach first."

"Good," I said, "but be assured that I'm willing to call Mike and I want to say to you that you cannot afford to allow the silence to continue. It's not healthy, it's not natural, it's not a healthy way for Mike to be responding to his unmet need for love. And you must not allow this pattern to get established in your relationship."

Two weeks later, I saw Jill at a public gathering, talking with some friends. She came over, smiled and said, "It worked. He started talking that same night. He told me how sorry he was that he had treated me so badly. He realized that was not a healthy way for him to respond and that he hoped that he would not do that again. I think I've got his love tank full, Dr. Chapman. I'm going to the beach next weekend. Mike has agreed and feels good about it."

"Have a great time," I said. I walked away with the confidence that Mike and Jill had learned a great deal about themselves and each other through their painful experience with the silent treatment.

One of the encouraging things about Jill and Mike's story is that Jill took positive action early in the marriage to deal with a silent partner. This was the first time Mike had ever treated her with silence for an extended period. She came for help and gained insight, understanding, and a strategy for dealing with the problem. Solving such problems early in marriage is always the ideal. Unfortunately, many couples have allowed the silent treatment to get entrenched in their relationship over many years of marriage.

The most common mistake of spouses who are married to non-communicating mates is to focus on the silence rather than on the reason for the silence. Mandy's husband, Brent, had never talked as much as she wished. Periodically, she would say to him, "I wish you'd talk more. I don't ever know what you're thinking. Just tell me what you want; don't just sit there." All of these statements struck deeply at Brent's self esteem. As a child he heard his mother tell others that her little boy was shy. He had felt inadequate about his lack of communication skills as long as he could remember. Now in marriage, his wife had picked up where his mother left off, thus confirming his feelings of inadequacy.

Mandy's focus is on Brent's silence. A much more productive route is to focus on why Brent is silent. She could say, for example, "I feel so frustrated by your silence and really would like to know what you are thinking. Did something happen at work, or did I say something?" If he says, "No, it's nothing like that," then at some point she should ask about his childhood—his parents, their comments, and his friends at school. Any of these could give her some real clues as to why Brent has developed a pattern of silence.

If she pursues questions about the family, Mandy will likely discover that Brent's mother spoke of him as shy and this set a pattern of Brent's perception of himself. Then she could express sympathy, opening the way for a dialogue. For instance: "I think I am beginning to understand why you don't talk as much as I talk. I can see how if growing up you had the perception that you were shy and silent that would definitely affect your talking patterns. I want you to know that I love you whether you talk or not. You are the man of my dreams. You have been such a wonderful husband. You have worked so hard to provide for us."

Such acceptance of his basic personality pattern and affirmation of his positive traits would likely begin to free Brent up to communicate more openly with Mandy. But as long as her statements are condemning, he will never talk more.

Not Just "A Male Thing"

I am often asked at my marriage seminars if it is a male thing not to talk. While it is true that most men talk less than most women, it is not true that men are the only noncommunicating spouses. I first met Wayne in Seattle, the city of eternal rain. He had on a tee shirt that said "You Can Tell When It's Summer in Seattle . . . The Rain Is Warmer." I laughed at his tee shirt, but I did not laugh at his story.

"Dr. Chapman, we've been married for five years now, and we've had a fairly good marriage. The only real problem is that Susan keeps everything inside and will not share with me her thoughts and feelings, especially if they are negative. I think it's because she grew up in a home where her thoughts and emotions were never welcomed. If she shared a negative emotion, she got a lecture on why she should not feel that way. If she shared her thoughts and they were different from her father's, she was told in no uncertain terms that she was wrong. As a result, she developed a pattern of holding her thoughts and feelings inside.

"I have tried to tell her that I am not her father. I consider myself a good listener. I do not get angry and scream at her. I've even taken some courses at church as a lay counselor, and I really would like to help her open up. But to this point, I have been unable to do so."

"Old patterns are hard to break," I said, "but I think you are moving in the right direction. She needs the assurance that you are there to listen, not to condemn." I asked if Susan was with him at the seminar.

"Yes," he said. "I'm really glad that she was willing to come."

FEAR OF EXPRESSING NEGATIVE FEELINGS AND THOUGHTS

"I'd like to meet her at the next break if possible," I said. When I saw Susan, I shared with her the gist of what Wayne had told me, to which she responded, "Dr. Chapman, I wish I could open up to Wayne. I really want to. I know it's important not only for him but for me. But I feel like when I share negative feelings and thoughts that it reveals that I am a bad person. I shouldn't have negative feelings, and I shouldn't think negative thoughts."

"What are the feelings that you have most difficulty sharing?" I asked.

"Anger is one," she said. "I wish I didn't get angry. Depression is another. Sometimes I feel so depressed; I hate myself when I feel that way."

I knew that Susan was active in her local church because Wayne had told me, so I said to her, "Did you know that Jesus often felt angry and that Jesus also felt depressed?" Susan looked shocked and said, "Really?"

"Yes," I said, "Anger and depression are common human feelings. They certainly do not mean that we are bad persons. Anger arises inside when we perceive that we or someone else has been treated unfairly. Anger reveals our concern for righteousness and justice. Anger is not wrong. The Bible says of God that He is angry with the wicked every day.[1] Jesus felt depressed hours before He went to the cross, but He did not allow His depression to control His behavior.[2] Negative emotions are not sinful," I said. "They simply reveal that we are humans and when we encounter certain situations in life, we feel depressed or sad.

"The important thing is that we do not allow our negative emotions to lead us to wrongful behavior. Sharing these emotions with Wayne or anyone is a positive part of the process of not allowing them to control our behavior. We process negative emotions by sharing them with a trusted friend. Emotions come and go. When we talk about them, they tend to go. When we hold them inside, they tend to stay."

Then I suggested to Susan what I've suggested to many people through the years.

"If you find it difficult to break the barrier of silence, try writing your thoughts and feelings in a letter to your spouse. Many times it is easier to write than it is to speak of such feelings. But as you become comfortable writing the letters and your spouse reads them with understanding and comfort and encouragement, you will eventually learn to verbalize your feelings and thoughts. Writing can be a big step in the process of learning how to openly communicate your inner self." Susan assured me that she would try this because she knew that it was important in her relationship with Wayne.

Six months later, I got a letter from Wayne telling me how thankful he was for my comments to Susan, that she had indeed started writing him letters almost immediately after the seminar and that now she was able to share verbally her thoughts and feelings with him. I wrote Wayne back and assured him that one of the reasons Susan was able to break this pattern of silence in her life was because he had demonstrated to her by words and actions the art of sympathetic listening. Had he on the other hand condemned her thoughts and feelings or gotten angry with her, she would have stopped the flow of words immediately.

Fear of the Spouse's Response

The reality is that many spouses have retreated to the den of silence because of fear of their spouse's response. I well remember the husband who said to me, "She's right. I don't talk. When I come home, I watch television or read the newspaper. And when my wife asks me to talk, I simply continue watching or reading. The reason," he said, "is that every time I share a thought or an idea, she pounces on it and tells me why I shouldn't think that way. If I comment on a newscast, she will always take the opposite side. If I make a comment about something that happened during my day and give my opinion on it, she rallies to the support of the other person.

"This has gone on ever since we got married. So I've decided it's safer not to talk. I can't take her constant disagreement with everything I say."

When I talked to his wife, her perspective was that her husband, who we'll call Lou, was dogmatic and opinionated and that most of the time his opinions were wrong. She was simply trying to help him see another perspective. She couldn't understand why he got so defensive when she disagreed with his ideas. She took that as immaturity and told him so. He had stopped talking because of fear that any comment that he made would stimulate what he considered to be an attack from his wife.

Later, as Lou and I talked further, I discovered that in childhood, he was never allowed to express his ideas. His parents had the philosophy "children are to be seen and not heard." Whenever Lou did share an idea, his father was quick to correct him.

Now as an adult, he had become a widely read person and felt that he had a rather good perspective on what was going on in the world. He prided himself in this knowledge. This had been his way of building his own self-esteem, seeking to overcome the negative messages he received from his father. When his wife disagreed with his ideas, it struck deeply at his self-esteem. That is why Lou became defensive and that is why he eventually stopped talking.

It took a while, but eventually we discovered that if his wife would frame her thoughts in the form of a question rather than a comment, Lou could receive it with less defensiveness. "What do you think about this perspective?" was easier for him to receive than for her simply to express the perspective as her own. After considerable counseling, Lou came to recognize that his wife's expressions of her ideas, though different from his, were not in fact designed to condemn him. He came to understand that people can have different ideas and still like each other. In fact, people do have different ideas. When we give people the freedom to disagree with us, we are giving them the freedom to be human. He was willing to talk again when he finally concluded that his wife was not against him. She just wanted the freedom to be a person and express her ideas even if they were different from his own.

BRINGING POSITIVE CHANGE:
MEET YOUR SPOUSE'S EMOTIONAL NEEDS

There are many reasons why some spouses become uncommunicative. Their unwillingness to share verbally finds its root in what is going on inside of them. Often it is unmet needs in the marital relationship that have stimulated resentment in the spirit of the silent spouse. His silence is a way of expressing this resentment. It is his/her way of saying, "I don't like you, so I will treat you as a non-person."

I don't mean that the silent partner is consciously thinking these thoughts; I mean these are the inner emotional reasons why he or she is not talking. If we can discover the emotions inside the person and the factors that give rise to these emotions, we are well on the way to helping the noncommunicating spouse to break his/her silence.

The spouse who seeks to be a positive change agent would do well to ask this question: "Does my spouse have an unmet emotional need that may be causing him to resent me?" The five needs which we discussed in chapter 5 are simply examples. They were: the need for love, freedom, significance, recreation, and peace with God. Thus each of us can ask ourselves the following:

- Does my spouse genuinely feel my unconditional love or has my love been conditional—I will love you if . . .
- Have I done anything to infringe upon my spouse's freedom? Does he feel that I am trying to control his life?
- Has my speech or behavior struck at her efforts to gain significance? Does she see me as condemning something that she values as being significant?
- Does he see me as a barrier to the fulfillment of his need for recreation and relaxation?
- Is my spouse struggling with the spiritual dimension of life? Does she see me as interfering with her search for peace with God?

Any one of these questions may uncover the source of your spouse's silence. The challenge then is to find a way to help him or her meet that emotional need and at the same time maintain your own integrity and get your own needs met.

CHANGE NEGATIVE PATTERNS OF COMMUNICATION

Another positive approach is to ask yourself, *Does my communication pattern make it difficult for my spouse to talk?* Negative communication patterns can silence a spouse. The solution is to change those patterns.

Here are some questions you can ask to determine whether your conversations with your spouse are negative:

- Do I often come across as complaining?
- Do I listen to my spouse when he talks, or do I cut him off and give my responses?
- Do I share how I would like things to be rather than complaining about how things are?
- Do I allow my partner space when he needs it, or do I force the issue of communication, even on those times when he needs to be alone?
- Do I maintain confidences or do I broadcast our private conversations to others?
- Do I openly share my own needs and desires in the form of requests rather than demands?
- Do I give my spouse the freedom to have opinions that differ from my own or am I quick to "set her straight?"

If you can answer yes to any of these questions, it may be time to change a negative communication pattern. Changing these patterns may be difficult, but it is the way toward loosening the tongue of a noncommunicative spouse.

DEVELOP LISTENING SKILLS

Developing the art of listening with the sincere desire to understand your spouse enhances the climate of open communication. There are many ways you can communicate "I care about what you say" just by listening. Give your spouse your undivided attention when he/she is talking; maintain eye contact when possible; turn off the TV, lay down the book or magazine, and give your mate your focused attention. All these actions communicate "Your words matter to me." To receive your spouse's ideas as information rather than an opinion that you must correct creates an atmosphere of acceptance. This doesn't mean that you agree with all of those ideas; it means that you give your spouse the freedom to hold those ideas.

Learning to control your anger and hear the person out also enhances communication. Loud, angry outbursts almost always stop the flow of communication. Practice "reflective listening," reflecting back the person's words in your own words. "Are you saying . . ." and "What I hear you saying is . . ." are phrases that help your spouse continue to clarify what he/she is saying. At times, indicate your understanding of the message: "I think I understand . . . I see what you're saying . . . That makes a lot of sense." Such statements tend to keep the spouse talking. All of us are more likely to communicate our inner thoughts and feelings if we believe that our spouse genuinely wants to hear what we want to say and will not condemn us.

Reality living reminds us that we cannot change our spouses, but we can influence them. To read or attend a course at a local college or church on the art of communication will be time well invested for the spouse who wants to be a positive change agent for a noncommunicating spouse. Your words, body language, and listening skills can have a profound positive or negative influence upon your spouse's freedom to communicate. If your spouse would join you in such a course or in reading a book, so much the better. But don't wait for him/her to join you. Take the initiative, go against your feelings if you must, but do something positive to enhance your own understanding of why people do not communicate. Obviously whatever you have tried in the past to help your spouse to communicate has not worked. It's time to take a new approach. You cannot make your spouse talk, but you can create a climate that is friendly to communication.

NOTES

1. Psalm 7:11, New International Version.
2. Matthew 26:37.

CHAPTER TEN

THE VERBALLY ABUSIVE SPOUSE

You are an imbecile. I don't know how anyone with your education could be as stupid as you are. You must have cheated to get your degree. If I were as stupid as you, I don't think I would get out of bed in the mornings." The words seemed to beat upon Betty incessantly. This wasn't the first time Betty had heard such insults from her husband, Ron. The tragedy was that she had come to believe them. She was suffering from severe depression that literally kept her in bed most days. She was the victim of verbal abuse.

We have long known the devastation of physical abuse in a marriage relationship. (The next chapter will discuss responses to that kind of abuse.) We are coming to understand that verbal abuse can be fully as devastating. Verbal abuse destroys respect, trust, admiration, and intimacy—all key ingredients of a healthy marriage.

Most of us "lose our temper" sometimes and may say harsh, cutting words that we later regret. But if we are spiritually and emotionally mature, we acknowledge that this is inappropriate behavior. We express sorrow and ask forgiveness of our spouse, and the relationship finds healing. The verbal abuser, on the other hand, seldom asks for forgiveness or acknowledges that the verbal tirades are inappropriate. Typically, the abuser will blame the spouse for stimulating the abuse. "She got what she deserved" is the attitude of the abuser.

Verbal abuse is warfare that employs the use of words as bombs and grenades designed to punish the other person, to place blame, or to justify one's own actions or decisions. Abusive language is filled with poisonous put-downs which seek to make the other person feel bad, appear wrong, or look inadequate.

The verbal bombardment can be stimulated by almost anything. A look, a tone of voice, a broken dish, or a crying baby can all pull the trigger on the arsenal of the verbal abuser. The verbally abusive spouse is out to punish, belittle, and control his partner, and he does it compulsively and constantly, showing little empathy for the feelings of the spouse.

Verbal abuse is a twentieth-century term but an ancient malady. Solomon, the wise king of ancient Israel, wrote "Do you see a man who speaks in haste? There is more hope for a fool than for him"; and "A fool gives full vent to his anger."[1] Solomon accurately understood the power of the tongue when he said, "The tongue has the power of life and death."[2] Indeed, abusive words can bring death—death to the spirit, and, if not corrected, death to the relationship. Those who have been verbally abused over long periods of time often say, "My emotions are dead. I used to feel hurt and anger; now all I feel is apathy."

Many abused spouses can identify with Judith who said to her divorce lawyer, "I never knew what to do. He would always notice little things and then fly off the handle. If he saw that I put the roll of toilet paper on the holder with the paper going over rather than under, he'd lose it. It was always silly things. I tried arguing, I tried crying, I tried threatening divorce. Nothing seemed to get his attention. He blamed me for everything. It was always my fault. He was perfect. I don't know what else to do."

Is there hope for Judith and thousands of other spouses who suffer the barrage of verbal attacks as a way of life? I believe there is, but that hope will not come in the form of a magic wand. It will be more like an exercise machine. It will require hard work and you must be consistent. Progress comes slowly, but your efforts will eventually be rewarded.

UNDERSTANDING THE SOURCE OF VERBAL ABUSE

Most people who practice verbal abuse as a way of life are suffering from low self-esteem. Emotionally, they are not the strong, confident, self-assured individuals they may appear to be. Inside they are like children trying desperately to become adults, fighting desperately but inappropriately to prove their worth. They are trying to bolster their own self-esteem by putting others down.

Many verbal abusers have an unconscious need to be seen as perfect. Social approval has become almost a holy quest for them. They often think that approval requires perfection. Thus, criticism jeopardizes approval. They explode at the slightest criticism because their self-worth is being threatened. That is why they must always win the argument; to acknowledge that they are less than perfect is to acknowledge their greatest fear—that they are, in fact, worthless.

The verbal abuser often grew up in a home with verbally abusive parents. He is expressing his anger in the same manner as his parents. His problem is compounded by his own stored anger often toward his parents but released toward his spouse. Any solution for the verbal abuser must address realistically the whole problem of how to manage anger.

LOVING SOLUTIONS:
1. AFFIRM THE NEED; REJECT THE BEHAVIOR

The spouse who would seek to redeem an abusing husband or wife must understand and accept the validity of the inner spiritual and emotional needs of the abuser. The inner need for self-worth, purpose, and fulfillment in life reflects our spiritual nature as people, and so the person needs to be affirmed. At the same time, we do not help an abuser by accepting his destructive efforts to meet these needs. Because we are so hurt by the verbal abuse, we often lash back in self-defense, and the need which gave rise to the verbal abuse goes totally unaddressed.

A better approach is to acknowledge your spouse's inner emotional needs and incorporate these in your response to his verbal abuse. After one harsh verbal attack, Marie said to Bob, "I know you must be terribly frustrated to speak to me in that manner. I wish you could share the pain that you feel inside. I know it must be intense to cause you to lash out at me so strongly. I would like to be a help to you, but I cannot help you when you express your hurt and anger in such destructive ways. If you could write me a note telling me what you feel and how strongly you feel it, maybe I could be there for you and could be the spouse you need." Marie was acknowledging Bob's inner struggles, but at the same time she was communicating that his verbally abusive behavior was inappropriate.

This healthy approach to verbal abuse is difficult for some wives because they have bought into their husbands' critical remarks, just as Betty had. The wife who has been ridiculed, threatened, told she is stupid, worthless, incompetent, a bad wife, and a poor mother may allow these messages to be self-fulfilling. As the verbal abuse increases, it is hard for her not to believe her husband. Eventually she may conclude that she does not deserve anything better and may give up any attempts to improve the situation. Her husband may tell her, "You ought to be thankful I keep you around because no one else would have you." She may come to believe what he says because there is no one else around to contradict his statements.

For this wife, the first step is to share her husband's abuse with a friend or counselor. She must first be able to reject these negative messages from her husband and rediscover her own self-worth. Only then can she become a positive change agent in the marriage. If she does not deal with her own damaged self-esteem, she will not have the emotional energy to take constructive action with her husband. This wife will need individual counseling before she is ready to implement the constructive suggestions found in this chapter.

2. Believe in the Worth of Your Partner

Behind every verbally abusive tongue is a person of value. In spite of her (or his) devilish ways, she bears the image of God and has innate value. It is this positive image which attracted you to your spouse before marriage. You saw something of value in his or her character and behavior. She met some of your own needs in the romantic stage of your relationship. Now it is time to remember that behind the facade of the verbally abusive lion to whom you are now married is the lamb which you used to cuddle. You married the lamb not realizing that the lion would emerge. Now you must believe that the lamb is still there, believe that with the help of God and others, the lamb can become predominant again. Your job is not to make the lamb return. Your job is to believe that it's there. It is the responsibility of your spouse to feed the lamb and starve the lion, but your belief in the existence of the lamb may encourage your spouse to do so.

On a quiet evening when Jeff had not yet unleashed a verbal attack, Marilyn said to him, "I've been thinking about us a lot the last few days. I've been remembering how kind you were to me when we dated. I'm remembering the tender touch, the kind words, the smiling face, the fun we had in those days. I guess that's why I believe in you so strongly. I know the good qualities that are there. Sometimes I lose that vision when I am hurt by your attacks, but I know the kind of man you are and I believe in that man. And I believe in my heart that the man I married is the man you really want to be. And I know that by God's help and your desire, you can reach that goal."

With those words, Marilyn is expressing belief in Jeff. She is giving him what all of us desperately want—someone to believe in us; someone to believe that we have good characteristics and that those good characteristics can flourish in our lives. Since the abuser is already suffering from low self-esteem, such comments build a positive sense of self-worth. If Jeff can come to believe in himself and believe that God's power is available to him, Jeff may well become the man that Marilyn remembers.

3. SHARE YOUR OWN FEELINGS

We do not help an abusing spouse when we act as though the harsh words do not hurt us. The answer is not to lash back, to retaliate with our own verbal abuse. The answer is to acknowledge that we have been wounded and need help. Your spouse needs to be reminded that you are also human and that abusive words cut deeply.

In the physical realm, there is a limit to the amount of pain one can endure before going to a physician. In the emotional sphere, the same is true. It is the inner pain from verbal abuse that pushes us to talk to a counselor, a minister, or a friend. But that pain should not be hidden from the spouse. He or she needs to live with an awareness that you are hurting and that your pain has led you to talk with someone. That fact may initially lead the spouse to further abuse, but ultimately it is a step toward healing.

In a contemplative mood, Mark said to Susan, "There is something I really need to share with you. It is not easy for me to say it, but my pain is forcing me to talk. Over the last several weeks, I've lived with a great deal of heartache. I tried not to express it in front of the children and up until now, I've chosen not to share it with you. But the verbal attacks that I have heard from you have brought me tremendous pain. I am not sure how I should respond. I know that some of the things you say are true, and I would really like to work on those things. I feel also that some of the things you have said were spoken out of anger and are exaggerated. But I want you to know that I can't go on hearing your verbal attacks week after week without going for help.

"I really want to have a positive relationship with you," Mark continued," but when I am hurting so deeply, it is hard to be responsive. I've made an appointment with a counselor. I don't know if you want to go with me or not but I feel that I must have some help. I believe in you and I don't think that your behavior over the last month is characteristic of the real you. At the same time, I can't bear the pain any longer."

Mark is on the road to help and perhaps Susan will join him.

4. AGREE ON A STRATEGY

Once the problem of verbal abuse is laid on the table, you must develop a strategy for responding to the verbal bombshells. If your spouse is willing, you may work out the strategy together; or if you are going for counseling, the counselor can help you work out a strategy. If your spouse is unwilling to go for counseling and unwilling to talk with you about the problem, you must work out your own strategy and announce it to your spouse. For example, Megan says to Barry in a context of calmness, "I want to share with you a decision I've made. As you know, I have talked with you in the past about how deeply I am hurt when you lash out at me with critical and demeaning remarks. It takes me days and sometimes weeks to get over the pain that I feel on those occasions. I have decided that the next time you lose your temper and begin to yell at me, I will take some time away from you in order to recover. I think my healing will be faster if we are apart.

"I wanted you to know what I am doing. I will not be abandoning you but I am trying to take constructive action to what has become a very destructive pattern in our relationship. I can't survive your attacks indefinitely. I don't believe that is the kind of person you want to be. I know there is another person inside of you and I believe in that person and I believe that with God's help, you will become the good person that you and I both know is there.

"I'm sharing this with you because I believe in you and I want you to know that I want to be as strong as I can to help you become the person you want to become."

Barry may immediately lash out, or he may be calm and express words of regret. Whatever his response, Megan will simply follow her plan the next time he explodes. Her time away with a friend or family member for two or three days will give him time to think and also help him realize the serious nature of his verbal abuse. She will repeat this strategy the next time he abuses her verbally.

If this strategy does not stimulate him to go for counseling, she will need to develop additional steps. It's important to have a plan and to follow the plan consistently.

Don't let verbal abuse "work." If the spouse gives in and does whatever the abuser is requesting, then the abuse is encouraged. We must never allow verbal abuse to work for the abuser. Typically, abusive patterns have succeeded in the past and that is why they become entrenched. If you decide not to let them work, you are taking a positive step in breaking the pattern. You could say to your spouse, "I have realized that in the past, I have encouraged your verbal outbursts by caving in to whatever you have desired of me. I realize now that this is wrong. I want you to know that in the future whenever you lash out at me in anger and verbally attack me, I will not be responsive to that kind of behavior. If you want to make a kind request of me as your spouse, I will certainly consider your request and may well do what you desire, but I will not encourage you to be a tyrant by giving in to you when you are ranting and raving." Having made such a statement, you must be consistent in following it.

THE POWER OF REALITY LIVING

Remember, reality number one in reality living requires that we take responsibility for our own attitudes. A verbally abused spouse must first of all refuse to believe the negative messages of the verbally abusing husband/wife. We must come to affirm our own worth in spite of the negative messages we are receiving from our spouses. Only as we come to see ourselves as persons of worth and value will we be able to take positive steps which have the potential of changing our marriage relationships. We recognize that we cannot change our spouse's verbal behavior, but we can influence that behavior.

Understand that verbal abuse reveals the abuser's own low self-esteem and his/her inability to handle anger in a constructive way. Then you are free to have more constructive responses to the abuser's verbal outbursts. We must understand that our own actions are not controlled by our emotions. Our own hurt, anger, or apathy may encourage us to give up, but we choose to take constructive action, thus moving against our negative emotions. We admit that we are not perfect nor have we been perfect husbands/wives, but our own imperfections do not mean that we are failures. Admitting our own failures, we are free to choose the high road of loving our spouses unconditionally.

Reality living also recognizes the power of love as an agent for good. (See reality number six in chapter 4.) Unconditional love means that I will treat my spouse with kindness and respect even though she is not reciprocating. Remember, love is not a feeling; it is an attitude with appropriate behavior. It is the attitude that says,

"I choose to look out for your interests. How may I help you?" This does not mean that love puts up with abusive behavior. Interestingly, even God in the New Testament Scriptures, while loving, chooses to discipline; in fact His love motivates Him to discipline His children.[3] Love sometimes must be tough. Love holds a spouse accountable for inappropriate behavior.

Love says, "I care about you too much to sit here and let you destroy me and yourself. I know that is not for your good and I will not cooperate in the process." Love takes constructive action for the benefit of the one loved regardless of how difficult the action may be.

Do the above suggestions guarantee that your spouse will change his or her abusive behavior? Unfortunately, no such guarantee can be given. We cannot determine another's choices. We can, however, make wise choices. We can be responsible people even when our spouse is being irresponsible. Remember, you are not responsible for your spouse's behavior. You are responsible for your own. You did not make your spouse a verbal abuser. You do choose what your response will be to that abuse. Retaliation (fighting fire with fire), capitulation (giving up and becoming a doormat), and denial (acting as though nothing is wrong) are all common responses to verbal abuse. None of them, however, is a healthy response.

Daniel, the Iowa pig farmer whom we met in chapter 1, is a good example of a verbally abused husband who practiced reality living. He is the one who said, "I consider myself a strong man. I don't usually let things get me down, but my wife's constant criticism has almost destroyed me. Other people can get on my case and I let it roll off like water off a pig's back, but when my wife constantly criticizes me it is like a dagger in my heart. She is such a negative person not only toward me but toward everyone and toward life in general. She stays depressed a lot of the time. . . . Her life is miserable and she tries to make my life miserable. I find myself wanting to stay away from the house and not be around her."

I met Daniel at one of my marriage seminars and after hearing his story strongly urged him to seek counseling on how he could be a constructive change agent in his marriage. He countered that the nearest counselor was fifty miles away. I assured him that it would be worth the drive. Two years later, I was greatly encouraged when I returned to Iowa for another marriage seminar and saw Daniel again. (He had driven 150 miles to attend the seminar.) This time his wife was with him, and at one of our break times he told me what had happened over the past two years.

A Pig Farmer's Discoveries

Daniel's first discovery in the counseling process was finding out why his wife's critical words had been so painful to him. Two factors gave him this insight. The first came from his family of origin. Daniel's family had also given him critical words. He could never do anything to his father's satisfaction. Thus, Daniel grew up with the feeling of inadequacy. As a boy, the record playing in his mind was, "When I get to be a man, I will be a success. I will prove my father wrong, and I will receive affirmation from my peers." In adulthood, Daniel had lived out that dream. His hard work and commitment had paid off; he was a successful farmer and was known not only in the county but in the state. He was indeed respected by his peers but the person whose affirmation he most desired, namely his wife, only echoed his father's condemning messages. What he had worked all his life to overcome was staring him in the face every day.

The second insight that helped Daniel understand himself was the discovery that his primary love language was words of affirmation. The thing that genuinely made him feel loved and appreciated was hearing affirming words. Thus, his wife was speaking a hostile, foreign love language as she gave him condemnation instead of affirmation. Her words stung more deeply because he was suffering from an empty love tank. Her critical words were like bullets piercing the tank itself. He was emotionally devastated.

Daniel also discovered something about his wife's needs. Debbie was operating out of her own unmet emotional needs. He learned her primary love language is quality time and that because of the long hours required on the farm and his strong desire to be a successful farmer, he had little time left over for her. In the earlier days of the marriage, Debbie had begged him to spend time with her, to take her to a movie, to attend the church picnic with her, to take a vacation in the summer, to spend two days in the city just having fun. But Daniel had been too busy for such "frivolous activities."

Now he realized that he had not spoken his wife's primary love language for years. He now realized that her critical words were desperate cries for love. Debbie's depression had grown out of her sense of hopelessness in the marriage, and her growing lack of interest in their sexual relationship was stark evidence that she felt little emotional love coming from him.

"With these insights," Daniel said, "I was able to take constructive action. I acknowledged to her that I was learning a great deal about myself and about marriage from my counselor. I told her that I recognized that in many ways I had not been a good husband and that with God's help I wanted to change that."

"She was shocked the morning I told her that I would like for us to go on a picnic at a nearby lake," he said. "She seemed almost incredulous. Nevertheless, when I came in from the morning chores and started taking a shower, she started packing the picnic. We spent three hours together, walking, sitting, and talking. I told her how sorry I was that I had spent so little time with her through the years and I wanted us to make the future different. She opened up and told me her pain from past years and reminded me of the times she had begged for my attention. Now I did not take these statements as critical but as genuine expressions of her need for love. Toward the end of the afternoon, we found ourselves hugging and kissing. It almost seemed like we were dating again."

Over the next couple of months, Daniel planned several other quality time experiences with his wife, and each evening he spent time talking and listening to her as they discussed the day's events. He noticed that Debbie was spending less time in bed each day and that her depression seemed to be lifting. She began to be more sexually responsive and in time, her whole countenance changed. The critical words stopped and after his wife read my book *The Five Love Languages,* she had recognized immediately that his primary love language was words of affirmation. It was now easy for her to give such words because her own love tank was filled by the quality time she had received from Daniel.

Debbie joined Daniel at the next marriage seminar and told me what the changes meant to her: "Daniel went for counseling and our marriage has totally changed. I am excited that we can come to the seminar together this year. I know that I am going to learn some things that will help both of us." The next day as she and Daniel left the seminar, she said, "Now I understand what happened to my husband last year. He got new hope for our marriage. I am so excited; I can hardly wait to get home and apply the things we've learned at the seminar."

Daniel and Debbie were on the road to marital growth primarily because Daniel had chosen the high road of reality living. In spite of his negative, hopeless feelings about his marriage, he had reached out for help, had changed his own attitude and behavior, and had become a constructive change agent in his marriage. He had discovered firsthand that although we cannot change our spouses, our positive actions can have a profound, positive influence on their behavior.

NOTES

1. Proverbs 29:20; 29:11, New International Version.
2. Proverbs 18:21, NIV.
3. Hebrews 12:5–7, NIV.

THE PHYSICALLY ABUSIVE SPOUSE

*D*omestic violence has become a problem of major proportions. Statistics on the reported cases of spousal abuse continue to escalate. Many police departments are overwhelmed by the number of calls related to physical abuse. Media focus has made physical abuse a matter of national concern. But for all the public attention given to this problem, the fact is millions of spouses continue to be abused every year.

The results of physical abuse are devastating not only to the one abused but also to the children who grow up in such homes. The results are often deadly.

Physical abuse is any act that inflicts bodily harm or is intended to do so. It may consist of hitting, shoving, kicking, choking, throwing objects, or the use of a weapon. The severity of physical abuse can range from a slap across the face to homicide. If verbal abuse can kill the spirit, physical abuse can eventually kill the person.

Sociologists have discovered certain patterns as to when and where spousal abuse occurs. The typical location of physical abuse is in the home, with the living room and the bedroom the most likely scenes of violence. The bedroom is the most likely place for a spouse to be killed. Marital violence is more frequent between the hours of 6 P.M. and midnight. Physical abuse usually is preceded by arguments. These arguments most often center around the management of children and disagreements over money. Violence is more likely to occur on weekends than on weekdays. As the frequency of physical abuse increases, the more severe are the attacks.[1]

THE CYCLE OF ABUSE

Research has shown a three-phase cycle in physical abuse.[2] First is the *tension building phase*. This is the period in which the abuser experiences a series of irritations. His frustration with them escalates and his feelings are held inside. As the feelings become more intense, he will verbally express his hostility. At this point, the wife may attempt to placate her husband, trying to calm him and avoid further confrontations. This may work temporarily, but the tension continues to build inside the abuser. The husband expresses further angry verbal responses. When the wife feels there is no hope of placating him, she tends to withdraw. The husband sees her withdraw and reacts with more intense anger. This phase of building tension may last anywhere from an hour to several months.

Next comes the *explosion phase*, when physical abuse actually occurs. The abuser now unleashes his aggressive behavior toward his spouse. This phase is ended when the battering stops. With it comes a reduction in the amount of tension.

The third phase is *remorse*. After the explosion, there is a period of relative calm. The abusive spouse may apologize profusely, show some kindness to the wife, and promise that the abuse will never happen again. Such behavior often comes out of a sense of guilt over the harm inflicted as well as fear of losing a spouse. During this phase, the abusive spouse may really believe that he will never, never express violence again. The partner often wants to believe him and thus remains in the relationship. During this "make up" time, the relationship may be better than at any other period in their lives; but eventually the abusive spouse will become irritated again. The tension will begin to build and the cycle will be repeated.

Beth said about her abusing husband, "He seems so sincere when he apologizes. He even has tears. He admits that what he did was wrong. He asks me to please forgive him and promises that it will never happen again. He seems so sincere I want to believe him, but every time it happens again." It was obvious that Beth wanted to believe her husband, but the reality was the abuse cycle was strongly established in his behavior.

LETTING THE ABUSE CONTINUE

In the vast majority of the cases, the wife is the one who is abused. There are cases where wives physically abuse husbands, but these are minuscule compared to wife abuse. And women typically let the abuse continue for months, even years. Research indicates that abused wives will be attacked, on average, thirty-five times before they finally call the police and press charges.[3] Why do battered wives wait so long to take action? Let's look at some of the common factors.

Typically the initial episodes of violence begin during the first year of marriage. In the beginning, the wife may blame herself, thinking that if she had acted differently her spouse would not have gotten violent. The first several episodes are infrequent. The husband is usually remorseful and the wife forgiving. As his explosions come more often, her belief in his apologies evaporates. Quite often by the time she realizes the abuse is serious, she feels overwhelmed and helpless. Many battered wives grew up in homes where there was a measure of physical violence. So in the early stages, she is somewhat accepting of her husband's abusive behavior. She may also suffer from low self-esteem acquired in her own childhood. If this is the case, she will tend to blame herself for her husband's explosions and she will seek desperately to meet his needs and to keep him happy.

Some battered wives are rescuers. They find their self-worth in helping those in need. Many wives of abusive husbands were first drawn to their spouses because of the man's need for someone to nurture him. The wife often enjoys the relationship when the abuse is not occurring. She bonds to the warmer side of her husband because he still meets some of her need to be loved.

Another reason why some abused wives procrastinate in taking action against their husband's abuse is that they have isolated themselves. Polly is a good example. When I asked why she had not shared this with her extended family, she said, "I didn't want them to know that we had problems. Before we got married, my mother told me that I should not marry Bill. I guess she saw something I didn't see. I was ashamed to tell her what was going on. I would stay away until my bruises healed; sometimes I didn't have contact with my family for weeks except on the phone. Polly also indicated that she had dropped out of her class at the local technical institute where she was trying to develop her computer skills. Her reasoning was the same—she didn't want anyone to know that she was having problems. Such isolation keeps the battered spouse from finding the help she needs.

Fear is another factor that keeps abused wives from taking actions. They know what their husbands have done in the past and they are afraid that if they contact family, a pastor, friend, or the police, the abuse will become even worse. These wives are often emotionally or economically dependent upon their husbands. After years of abuse, they have little self-confidence. Their security is in the familiar. The prospect of disrupting family life and the security is more than they can bear. They also may depend upon their husbands for finances. Even if they are working outside the home, chances are they do not believe that they could live on their salary. Thus their emotional or economical dependency on their husbands keeps them in the prison of fear.

I first met Jennifer a year before she married Mitch. She was a happy though timid twenty-one year old. She came to me to discuss her problems with self-esteem. She had fallen in love with Mitch although her family did not particularly care for him. She admitted that he was sometimes "rather blunt," but she understood that "it was just his way." She wanted desperately to get married and believed that Mitch was her man. After marriage, they moved rather soon out of town where Mitch secured a better job. Ten years later when I encountered Jennifer at one of my marriage seminars held in her city, she was a young mother riddled with fear. She told me her story of physical abuse so severe that she had been to the hospital emergency room three times in the last two years. Her parents knew nothing of what was going on. She did not have a job and had no friends. Financially she saw no hope of making it without Mitch. She was virtually a prisoner in her own house, feeling desperate and helpless. Many battered spouses can identify with Jennifer.

Is there hope for the thousands of Jennifers who suffer physical abuse from their husbands? Does reality living offer any genuine hope? I believe the answer to those questions is yes. An abused wife can become a positive change agent in the marriage, but I do not believe that she can do it alone. She will need the help of a trained counselor, the support of family or friends, and she will need to draw upon her spiritual resources. Let me illustrate by sharing the story of Mitzi, who found reality living restored not only her life but her marriage.

Reality Living: Mitzi's Story

Mitzi, you may remember, was sitting in my office wearing dark glasses and a long-sleeved sweater in mid June. She removed her sunglasses and revealed her blackened eye, the result of her latest violent episode. When she removed her sweater, her arms were blue from bruises inflicted by her enraged husband, Bruce.

"Dr. Chapman, I've got to have help," she said. "My husband lost control. He hit me with the telephone repeatedly and he threw a Coke bottle at me. I can't live like this." When I asked if anything like this had happened before, she responded, "Yes, several times, but I've never shared it with anyone until now. . . . This time is the worst and I know that I can't take any more chances. I should not have let it go on this long. I need help in deciding what to do."

In further conversation with Mitzi, I discovered that she grew up in a home where her father was physically abusive to her mother. Mitzi had never been physically abused by her father, but she had suffered much verbal abuse. She still remembered the day her father told her that she was a loser, that she was just like her mother, and that he pitied the man who would marry her. Now I understood why for the first twelve years of their marriage, Mitzi had taken Bruce's abuse as something she deserved. She was living out the prophecy that her father had made.

Mitzi had told no one about the abuse because of fear. She feared telling her parents because she didn't want to hear her father say, "You got what you deserved." And she knew in her heart that her mother had no answers to physical abuse. She feared telling her employer, thinking she might lose her job. She feared telling friends at church, ashamed of what was going on in her home. Now this most recent episode, the most violent of all, had finally pushed her to reach out for help.

She entered my office convinced that divorce was her only hope, yet she saw no way to leave Bruce. She knew that financially she and her six-year-old son could not live on her salary. She knew that asking her parents for financial assistance would reap her nothing but condemnation. She saw no way to survive apart from Bruce yet she knew that she could not endure further abuse. She feared that if she left, Bruce would kill her or harm their son. Mitzi exhibited many of the common characteristics of an abused wife: low self-esteem, isolation, a sense of helplessness, fear, and financial dependence upon her husband.

As a counselor, I knew that these issues had to be dealt with before Mitzi would have the emotional strength to take positive action in her marriage. I hoped that we could make some progress in these areas before the next violent episode erupted. Mitzi indicated that usually after the explosion, things would be rather calm for two or three months before Bruce exploded again. I told Mitzi that I would be willing to help her if she would make a commitment to work with me for one year and to the best of her ability do the things that I recommended. "Dr. Chapman, I'm willing to do anything," she replied. "I've got to have help."

I made three requests of Mitzi that first session. First, I asked that she agree to meet with me once a week for the next three months while we worked on helping her get to the place where she could take some constructive action in her marriage. Second, I asked her to begin attending the next week a local spouse abuse support group. I knew that here she would learn to tell her story to others and find encouragement from a supportive group. I knew also that in the group she would learn about the local shelter for battered women and would know that if there were a crisis, she would have a place to go twenty-four hours a day. Finally, I requested that she read the book *Search for Significance*,[4] which deals with understanding the basis of self-esteem. She agreed and consistently followed through with all three requests.

By the end of the three months, Mitzi was coming to see herself in a totally new light. She recognized that she was a person of worth, that she had average intelligence, was as capable as the next person, and was coming to understand that she was responsible for her own attitudes and behavior and that while she could not change Bruce's behavior, she could influence his behavior by her own actions. She was also coming to understand that while verbalizing her emotions to me and her support group was extremely important, her behavior need not be controlled by her emotions. Even with feelings of fear, she could still take positive actions. In short, she had laid the foundation for reality living.

According to Mitzi, Bruce had been rather calm during the first two months following the last explosion. But the third month, she was beginning to feel the tension building within Bruce. He was becoming more and more verbally critical of her and would get upset at the smallest irritation. We both felt that the possibility of another explosion was imminent. I felt it was time for Mitzi to take the "tough love" approach to Bruce's abusive behavior. Some of Mitzi's fears resurfaced. "I know in my heart that you are right," she said, "but I'm still fearful of what he will do."

I was sympathetic with her fear because I knew that it was based in reality. There was every possibility that if she took action to seek to influence his behavior, he was likely to be physically violent. However, if she took no action, he would also be physically abusive. We both agreed that the tough love approach was better than the "wait and get hit" approach.

In the support group, Mitzi had met a lady who was separated from her husband and looking for a roommate with whom she could share the rent. After talking with the support group leader, I agreed with Mitzi that this was a good place for her to stay, at least for a few weeks or months. I suggested that she write a letter to Bruce telling him her pain and frustration from the past abuse and letting him know that she loved him too much to remain in the relationship and let him destroy her and ultimately himself; that she had decided that the best thing for her to do was to move out until he could find an answer to his abusive explosions. The letter would indicate her willingness to work on their marriage after he had extensive counseling to help him learn how to deal with his anger and frustration; but until he got such help, she could no longer stay in the home.

Mitzi wrote the letter. At the end of the letter, she noted that if he wanted counseling, she would suggest that he call my office and she gave him the phone number. Friends in the support group agreed to help Mitzi move her things out of the house, and she left him the letter on the kitchen table.

Bruce's response was immediate. Before my secretary arrived in the office the next morning, he had left a message on her voice mail asking for an appointment with me. Four days later, he was in my office. He was angry, remorseful, frustrated, and "willing to do anything to get Mitzi back." I told Bruce that I was glad he had come to see me. I told him that I hoped that his dream of Mitzi's coming back could someday be realized, and I told him that I believed Mitzi was open to that. I also told him that this would not happen next week or next month. I told him that I was proud of Mitzi for the actions she had taken, that I thought it was a genuine expression of her love for him, and that if he loved her and wanted his marriage to be restored, he would have to do the hard work of learning how to deal with anger and how to love her more effectively.

"That process will take weeks and maybe months," I said, "but if you're willing, I'd be glad to refer you to a colleague who specializes in helping men like you. I will keep in touch with the counselor and whenever the counselor feels that it's time to talk about reconciling the marriage, I will be happy to work with you and Mitzi on that process."

Then I warned Bruce that any effort to contact Mitzi or to be physically abusive to her would jeopardize his possibility of restoring their relationship. "This is a time not for retaliation but a time for personal growth in your life," I suggested. "The counselor I would refer you to has a support group for men who have physically abused their wives. Become a part of that group, Bruce. I believe your progress will be faster if beyond individual counseling you participate with the group." I knew that my colleague would suggest this but I wanted to plant the seed in Bruce's mind so he would have time to think about it.

The next week Bruce began his counseling, and the following week he enrolled in the support group. He was not 100 percent successful in following my suggestion that he make no contact with Mitzi for at least a month. Three times in the first month, he tried to make contact with her. Once he tried to call her at her work; once he was in the parking lot when she got off from work and tried to talk to her. Fortunately, she had a friend walking with her to the car and he did not make contact although she saw him and he saw her. His third attempt was to show up at her office, which created somewhat of a scene until he was asked to leave by her supervisor. Each of these incidents was reported to me by Mitzi; I in turn shared these with Bruce's counselor. The counselor confronted Bruce and affirmed that this was not the way to restore his marriage, that in due time we would arrange for him to have a conversation with Mitzi; but he needed to concentrate on his own personal growth and understanding.

Over the next four months, Bruce's counselor and support group helped him to understand that expressing anger in an abusive manner is a learned behavior and that it can be unlearned; that he must take responsibility for his violent outbursts; that such outbursts are never constructive; and that he must learn constructive ways to process his anger. Bruce also began to recognize that violence is never justified in a marriage and that uncontrolled expressions of anger must be stopped if the marriage is to continue. He learned how to recognize when tension is building up inside and how to process minor irritations before they get to the explosive state.

Bruce came to understand that much of his behavior was motivated by his own low self-esteem and was, in fact, an effort to prove his worth, but that such efforts were never successful and that each explosion led to a greater sense of incompetence. He learned and practiced with his support group methods for resolving conflict and was assured that he need not continue in his abusive behavior.

The basic goal in treating abusive spouses is not to eliminate anger but to replace abusive expressions of anger with positive expressions. One advantage of group therapy is that group members tend to confront each other more directly and perhaps more effectively than the therapist. Having other men in the group who say "I don't like what I'm doing and I want to stop" is a powerful model for the abuser. The group experience also helps men overcome some of the emotional isolation from other men. After a group is established, members often will reach out to other members during times of crisis. Such a support group serves for the abusing husband much the same role as an Alcoholics Anonymous group does for the alcoholic.

RETURNING HOME

After several weeks, Bruce's counselor arranged for a joint meeting with Bruce and Mitzi. The discussion, however, was not related to restoring their marriage. The session dealt with how they had handled anger in the past and how they anticipated handling anger in the future. In this session, Mitzi assured Bruce that if he could learn to handle his anger and they could learn how to love and support each other, she was willing to discuss the possibility of restoring their marriage. This gave Bruce the needed encouragement to continue the counseling process. For most men, the strongest external motivator to get counseling is the desire to keep their wives. This is often the only way that men will reach out for counseling. Their wives have said, "You participate in counseling or else." Eventually the motivation will be internalized in a sincere desire to change what the abuser realizes is inappropriate behavior. Few abusing husbands will go for counseling without such pressure. It is important that the wife not return to the home too soon and thus remove this strong motivator for him to continue counseling.

It was nine months after Bruce started his counseling that we all agreed that it was time to begin marriage counseling. I began seeing Bruce and Mitzi weekly for one month, and bimonthly for the next two months. At the end of three months of marriage counseling, we agreed it was time for Mitzi to move home. She had been away for a little over a year. During the three months I was counseling with this couple, they had a dinner date once a week. Thus, Mitzi had not only our counseling sessions to give her confidence but the realization that she could be with Bruce alone and they could talk without angry outbursts. She moved back home with confidence and I continued to counsel with them every two weeks for the next three months, and once a month for the following six months. During this time, Bruce and Mitzi attended a three-month marriage enrichment clinic offered by a local church which met once a week and had homework assignments. They both realized that a happy marriage is something that requires regular attention, and they committed themselves to a pattern of growth.

My last session with Bruce and Mitzi was eight years ago, but I have continued to keep in contact with them from time to time. They have consistently followed two suggestions that I gave in our final session. One was to attend a marriage enrichment event every year. Some years this is a weekend retreat; other years, this is a class that runs for six or eight weeks. And the second suggestion was to read and discuss a book on marriage once a year. These are two practical ways for keeping a healthy marriage invigorated. In the eight-plus years that Bruce and Mitzi have been back together, Bruce has never physically harmed Mitzi. They have had the normal misunderstandings and conflicts which they have had to process. Sometimes they have each raised their voices and felt anger toward each other, but they have learned how to call "time out" until the anger subsides and they can resolve the conflict.

The fact that they both dealt responsibly with the problem of physical abuse and have learned how to relate to each other in a healthy manner has built up self-esteem in both of them. Bruce and Mitzi have shared with friends that the crisis centering around his physical abuse has been the biggest learning experience in their lives. Both of them shudder to think what might have happened if Mitzi had not taken the tough love approach in response to Bruce's abuse. They now lead workshops on anger management in a marriage enrichment class sponsored by their church. Who could be more qualified to lead such a group?

THE PRINCIPLES IN ACTION

Let me briefly summarize how Mitzi applied the principles of reality living. First of all, she recognized that she is responsible for her own attitude. Before counseling, her attitude was "I am in an abusive marriage and my only hope is divorce." In counseling, her attitude shifted to "I am in an abusive marriage, and I will use this to gain self understanding." Later her attitude became "I understand why I have been passive in dealing with my abusive husband. I will now seek to discover positive actions." She came to understand that she could not change Bruce's behavior but that there were positive actions she could take which held the potential for influencing his behavior. She understood that her negative emotions need not control her actions. She took positive actions even when she had feelings of fear and uncertainty. Such actions did, in fact, have a positive effect on Bruce's behavior. They motivated him to get the counseling he needed to gain the self-awareness and understanding necessary to make positive changes in his life. Mitzi demonstrated that love is the most powerful weapon for good in the world, even if that love must be tough love. Together, she and Bruce learned how to help meet each other's emotional needs for love, freedom, significance, self-worth, recreation, and eventually peace with God.

Reality living with an abusive spouse does not always produce such satisfying results, but it does always stimulate growth in the life of the person who chooses to practice it. I want to say once again I do not believe that a spouse who has been abused over a long period of time will be able to take such constructive actions without the help of professional counseling. I urge you if you are in an abusive marriage to seek such counseling immediately. It will be worth the time, effort, and money you spend and offers the greatest potential for a positive outcome in what has become a destructive marriage.

NOTES

1. M. A. Straus, R. J. Gelles, and S. K. Steinmetz, *Behind Closed Doors: Violence in the*

America Family (Garden City, N.Y.: Anchor, 1980), 31–50.

2. Lenore Walker, *The Battered Woman Syndrome* (New York: Springer, 1984), 95–96.

3. E. Carpenter, "Traumatic Bonding and the Battered Wife," *Psychology Today* (June 1985), 18.

4. Robert S. McGee, *Search for Significance* (Houston: Rapha, 1990).

THE SEXUALLY ABUSED/ ABUSIVE SPOUSE

met Justin during a weekend marriage enrichment retreat held in the beautiful Colorado Rockies. He was an outdoorsman and seemed full of life. But behind closed doors, he shared his heart.

"Dr. Chapman, my wife and I have been married for fifteen years now and we have a fairly good marriage. She's a good woman and a good mother, but there's one area of our marriage that we've never been able to solve. My wife has almost no interest in sex. In fact, she is fairly resistant to any sexual desire that I express. She says that she just doesn't feel comfortable with anything sexual. She won't even allow me to fondle her breasts. Dr. Chapman, is that normal?"

I could tell that Justin was hurting deeply. I cut to the heart of the matter with my next question. "Do you know if she was sexually abused as a child?" He nodded his head and said, "Yes. That all came out several years ago. She shared it with me and then with our pastor. We prayed about it, and I think she forgave her father. We didn't talk about it much after that." Justin and his wife were experiencing the painful residue of the sexual abuse of children.

Unfortunately, thousands of couples can identify with their problem.

Sexually abused children eventually become adults. Many of them will marry and discover that time did not heal the scars. In this chapter we will walk behind closed doors and observe two painful realities related to sexual abuse: first, the pain of living with a spouse who was sexually abused as a child; and second, the pain of discovering that your husband has sexually abused your children. In both situations emotions run deep, and pain lingers long. Answers seem elusive and frustration often reigns. Sexuality is at the heart of our humanity and when it is distorted in childhood, it poisons the root systems of our relationship skills as adults.

Can "reality living" help us untangle the twisted wires of sexual identity and find marital intimacy? I believe the answer is yes, but the process will take time, patience, and most likely the help of a professional counselor. Reality living begins with the affirmation that sexual abuse is morally wrong and has devastating emotional and physical effects upon the person who is abused. By sexual abuse I mean any sexual activity, verbal or physical, which is forced upon another individual without his/her consent, which uses his/her as an object to meet another person's sexual desires. Such an act perpetrated upon a child sets in motion a whole series of emotional and physical reactions that have a detrimental effect upon a child's normal sexual maturation process.

This distortion of sexuality follows the child to adulthood and often causes problems in the marital relationship. These victims of sexual abuse will often find it extremely difficult to enjoy healthy sexual interaction with their spouses. Many are filled with shame, guilt, fear, anger, and often a revulsion toward sex. These deep-seated emotions are often accompanied by the inability to enjoy kissing, touching of breast or penis, and often an aversion to looking at a naked body, including one's own. The person does not desire to have these negative emotions related to sexual matters but finds it impossible to feel differently. Thus, we are dealing with an extremely serious roadblock to a physically intimate marriage.

Let's explore the kind of steps that can be taken to help a couple navigate beyond this sexual roadblock and find the intimacy they both desire. We also will look at how to deal with a sexually abusive spouse as we revisit Robbie, the mother who discovered her husband had abused their two daughters earlier in their marriage. There are lasting, loving solutions when we understand motives and apply the principles of reality living.

CONSEQUENCES OF SEXUAL ABUSE: MIXED FEELINGS TOWARD SEX

Often the sexual abuses of childhood are well hidden by the person. In fact, the wife or husband of an abused spouse may not even suspect it. Let's return to Justin.

"Were you aware of the fact that your wife had been sexually abused by her father before you were married?" I asked Justin during a break at the Rocky Mountain seminar.

"No," he said, "and that's a part of what bothers me. Before we were married, she seemed to be sexually responsive. In fact, we were sexually active before we got married. It was a year or two into the marriage before she started drawing back from sexual involvement. If the sexual abuse was the problem, I don't understand why she could have been sexually responsive before marriage and in the early days of our marriage. That's why I've never felt that was the problem."

I shared with Justin that one of the common characteristics of females who have been sexually abused is that in adulthood they often have ambivalent feelings toward sex. At times, they can feel that the only way to be loved is to be sexually active. Sometimes they are active with several partners but at other times, they draw back from sex and want nothing to do with it. In marriage, this ambivalence can be very frustrating. On a given day, she may make comments which lead him to believe that she is interested in being sexually intimate. She may even flirt with him, but when it comes to the actual time of foreplay and intercourse, she becomes a stone. "Yes," he interrupted, "that's exactly the way she is some days."

"Victims of sexual abuse often suffer from bouts of depression in which they withdraw not only from sex but from life itself," I continued. Justin was nodding yes. "They often suffer from low self-esteem and will make negative comments about themselves. Seldom expressed but often felt is a sense of hopelessness—that life will not get better and in fact, 'I do not deserve a good life.' Shame and guilt from the sexual abuse is often borne by the victim. Victims feel guilty even though the abuse was not their fault. What your wife has inside is a lot of mixed emotions and many false ideas about what has happened to her and the results—thoughts such as 'I'm a failure; I can never be close to anyone; people will betray you; my body is ugly; sex is something that is taken from you; I'll never be able to forgive my father and I'll never be able to forgive myself.'

"These false impressions, coupled with the emotions of guilt, shame, betrayal, and sometimes denial have held her in bondage for many years. It is like a cancer eating away at her emotional, spiritual well-being. She will not be healed without help," I suggested.

I could tell that what I was saying made sense to Justin, and he was beginning to realize that he had underestimated the impact of his wife's sexual abuse on her behavior throughout their marriage. I said, "The devastating results of sexual abuse are seldom ever removed by one visit to the pastor. That is a starting place, but it is only the first step of many which must be taken. If your wife is to find healing from the pain of sexual abuse and if the two of you are to find sexual intimacy, she will need your support, God's help, and the guidance of a caring counselor. Few people ever find genuine healing without these three ingredients."

I gave Justin the name of a counselor near his hometown and suggested that if his wife were willing, they should initiate the counseling as soon as possible. Justin was ready, and he hoped that his wife would be willing.

After the break, the seminar resumed. When we came to the section on sexual intimacy, I noticed that Justin's wife seemed somewhat uncomfortable. But at the end of the session, she sought me out and asked the simple question, "Dr. Chapman, is there any hope for someone who has been sexually abused as a child? I want to experience the kind of positive sexual relationship that you described, but it seems almost impossible."

I tried to communicate my sympathetic feelings for her struggle. Having worked with so many people in her situation through the years, I know that it's easy to lose hope. I assured her that there could be healing for past pain and that she could grow to have a healthy sexual relationship with her husband. I recommended a book, *Beyond the Darkness: Healing for Victims of Sexual Abuse,*[1] and told her that most people would need counseling to find ultimate healing.

Two years later, I was encouraged when I got a letter from Justin telling me that he and his wife had read the book, discussed it together, and agreed to seek counseling. "It has been the greatest learning experience of our lives," he said. "Neither of us knew anything about the impact of sexual abuse. I am saddened to think that my wife suffered silently from the pain of being betrayed by her father for all those years. I realized that I had focused on my own disappointment in our sexual relationship and had not understood the impact of the abuse upon her."

RECALLING THE PAST

Justin indicated that at first, his wife was reluctant to share all the details of her abuse with the counselor. She didn't want to dig back into the pain of those experiences, but the counselor had assured her that this was necessary for genuine healing, and that what had happened for so many years was that the pain had been covered up by pretense. That pain had never been extracted, the counselor said, and talking about it in the counseling setting was the best way to extract it and find genuine healing. The counselor had helped his wife understand that her father was responsible for this act, that as a child, none of the responsibility was hers. With the counselor, she came to understand and work through her many conflicting emotions about her father. Since her father was deceased, the counselor helped her symbolically confront her father with what had happened. The counselor had helped Justin understand how to be supportive of his wife as she sought inner healing and how to be patient with her as she developed a healthier perspective on sex.

In Justin's own words, "Beginning with holding hands and progressing to warm hugs, we have moved down the road. I have tried not to push her and to be understanding when the progress sometimes seemed slow. I now feel that we are genuinely beginning to express love to each other sexually. I believe that things will get better as we continue to learn and grow. I just wanted you to know that your seminar was the beginning of our healing." Justin's letter is the kind of encouragement that keeps marriage enrichment leaders motivated.

I want to make several observations about the progress that Justin and his wife made. First, progress comes as the couple begins to *take sexual abuse seriously.* Whitewashing the problem will never remove the distorted emotions. Second, both partners must *be willing to break the silence and talk to someone outside the marriage about the problem.* Justin's wife had tried this several years earlier when she shared her history with Justin and together they shared it with a minister. But the process was frustrated when there was no follow-through.

Problems related to sexual abuse are seldom solved unless a couple reaches out for help, which leads me to the third observation: *a trained counselor can have a key role.* Few couples will find lasting answers to the fallout of sexual abuse without the help of a trained professional. Reading good books on the subject can get one started in the right direction, but true healing requires the help of a fellow human being who can hear the pain, empathize with the hurt, and give understanding and guidance.

THE SEXUALLY ABUSED MAN

Victims of sexual abuse are not limited to the female gender. Research is indicating a growing number of young men who were sexually abused as children or young teens experience sexual dysfunction years later in their marriages. Perhaps you remember Betsy, whom we also met in chapter 1. She had been married for six years when she came to my office for counseling, complaining that her husband had not been sexually intimate with her during their entire six years of marriage. Puzzled that her husband had no apparent interest, she told me frankly, "I want to have intimacy in my marriage, and I don't want to leave my husband, but I don't know what to do. We've talked about it a few times and he's told me not to worry about it, but I do worry about it. It's just not right. Something is wrong and I don't know what to do about it."

In coming to me, Betsy was taking the first step in reality living. She was going against her emotions of fear in reaching out for help. I commended her for taking this brave step and assured her that I would help her take additional steps in her efforts to be a positive change agent in her marriage. During our ensuing dialogue, she recounted their relationship before marriage.

"We met only a year before we got married. He is the only man I ever really loved. Before marriage, I didn't see anything that caused me to question his sexuality. He hugged and kissed me with passion. We never had sexual intercourse and I was grateful that he never pushed me in this way. It was one of the things that I respected about him."

"After marriage, did he continue to kiss and hug you?" I asked.

"Yes, for a while. But we never had intercourse. He always said, 'Let's take it slow.' That was fine with me at first, but it never went beyond hugging and kissing and eventually even that stopped. In other ways, Dr. Chapman, he's a wonderful husband. He's a hard worker, he treats me with kindness and respect, we enjoy doing things together. We really have a good marriage except for this one area."

"After six years of marriage," I said, "I think it's rather obvious that this problem is not going to take care of itself, and I think you are wise to be reaching out for help. However, we can't get very far without your husband's cooperation. I want to suggest that you go home and within the next two or three days, tell your husband that you've been thinking a lot about your marriage and that in many ways, he is the most wonderful husband you could imagine. Give him positive affirmation for his good qualities but also tell him that you are very disappointed in the sexual part of your marriage and that you have decided that you are going for counseling to try to find out how you can cope with the situation and that you would like to invite him to go with you."

"He won't go," she blurted out. "I've asked him before. I know he won't go for counseling."

"I'm sure you are right, but he can't keep you from going. What you are doing is informing him of the steps that you are taking. He can never say that you went behind his back. You are telling him your motivation up front. You are probably right; he will not be willing to come with you. At any rate, call my office and make another appointment. Let him know when you are seeing me and again invite him to go with you. If he is still unwilling, then you come alone. Now he knows that you have come to see me. It will give me the freedom to call him after our next session and let him know that you have shared with me something of the problem in your marriage. I can assure him that you seem to be sincere in your efforts of wanting to deal with the problem, but I cannot help you without at least having one session with him to find out his perspective on the problem. Most of the time when I call husbands in this situation, they will agree to come in for at least one session."

She agreed to our strategy and that is, in fact, what happened. Her husband, Brent, was unwilling to come with her, but he did come to see me alone. In the first session, he poured out his story of sexual abuse as a child by a favorite uncle and later by a cousin. This got him involved in a homosexual lifestyle during high school with several different partners, he explained. In college, he had both homosexual and heterosexual relationships. In fact, he became obsessed with sex and flunked out of college after his second year. Shortly thereafter, he had a religious conversion. Brent's overt sexual behavior changed almost instantly but his internal fascination with sex led him to obsessive masturbation.

When he met Betsy at church, he was enamored to think that a girl of her stature and purity would be interested in him. Of course, she knew nothing of his past sexual lifestyle and he was not about to tell her for fear that he would lose her. In building his relationship with Betsy before they were married, Brent became emotionally revolted by his own earlier lifestyle and wished that he was as pure as she. Sex became almost a devil to him and he came to hate his own sexuality. In fighting this personal, emotional warfare against his past failures, he became impotent.

This impotence alleviated his temptation to be sexually active with Betsy before marriage but after marriage, it also rendered him incapable of having normal sexual relationships with Betsy. Brent had hoped that the problem would soon go away and Betsy would never have to know of his struggle. The problem had not gone away, however, and in coming to see me, he was sharing his story for the first time.

Revealing the Past

Because of his openness, I knew that Brent was on the road to recovery. It often takes numerous counseling sessions for a man to reveal what Brent had revealed to me in our first session. I told him how grateful I was that he had chosen to see me and how encouraged I was that he was so open. I assured him that this was the first step toward healing. I told him that I thought his wife would be supportive and I believed that, with counseling, the problem could be solved.

I asked him if he would be willing to come with her the next time and in my presence share with her something of what he had shared with me. He said that he would but that it would be the hardest thing that he had ever done in his life. "That's probably true," I said, "and one of the best things you've ever done in your life." I later called Betsy and asked if I could see her briefly the day before our counseling session together. She agreed. I tried to prepare her for what she was going to hear and told her how happy I was that her husband had chosen to share these things with me and was now willing to share them with her. I did not reveal the content, but I told her that what she would hear would make her very sad and perhaps stimulate anger and other emotions inside of her.

I knew that Betsy had a strong faith and I suggested that she pray that God would give her the ability to accept the truth and the strength to work through the problems. I told her that I felt that she was a key element in Brent's being willing to be open with me and that I believed with her support, he would take the necessary steps to find healing.

The next session went as I had hoped. Brent was open; he told his wife about his past homosexual involvement. He expressed deep guilt and he told Betsy that if she could no longer accept him, he would understand. Betsy said with tears, "I am deeply disappointed, but I love you. And I will stick with you and with God's help, we will find an answer to this problem." She did. And they did.

In the following weeks, I counseled with Brent weekly. We walked through his past. With great strength but not without fear, he confronted those who had originally abused him. They did what typically happens—denied that they had done anything wrong. But in confronting them, Brent assured his own healing. Releasing them to God, he also released his resentment and recognized that in spite of what they had done to him as a child, he could now as an adult find healing. After our first two sessions, I met again with Betsy and told her that I thought that within the next few weeks, her husband would begin to reach out to her with physical touch. I encouraged her to be responsive to his initiatives but not to push anything, to let him move at his own pace. Within three weeks, he was indeed reaching out to hold hands as they watched television together. And a week later, he embraced her and kissed her passionately. Within three months, the impotency was gone. At that juncture, I began marriage counseling with them for several sessions, helping them look at their entire relationship and develop positive ways of communicating with each other.

Once the sexual barrier was overcome, they progressed rapidly. For several years now, they have had what they both consider to be a normal sex life. Betsy's only regret is that she did not reach out for help much sooner.

Sexual abuse as a child greatly impacts every victim. It distorts the emotions and thoughts related to one's sexuality. These distortions will differ with each victim because of our unique personality differences, but the answer lies in facing the issue squarely and getting the needed help. Victims who are willing to accept reality living will acknowledge their own failures without taking on the responsibility for the original abuse. They will come to recognize that their thinking and their emotions are distorted and they will go against their feelings of fear and shame and reach out to find help. A supportive spouse will be a great asset in this journey toward healing and the spouse must often be the one who initiates the process which eventually leads the victim to help.

When Your Husband Sexually Abuses Your Children

Before we leave the subject of sexual abuse, I want us to revisit Robbie, who attended one of my seminars in Birmingham. Tears flowed freely as she said, "I discovered recently that my husband has sexually abused both of our daughters. One is now sixteen and the other is eighteen. Apparently this has gone on for several years, but I didn't know it until about a month ago. My older daughter finally went for counseling on her college campus; that's what brought it all out. Then she talked with my younger daughter and found out that the same thing had been happening to her. As soon as I heard it, I took my daughter and went to live with my mother. Right now, I hate him and never want to see him again."

I found out that she had only talked with her husband once since she left. He told her that he knew what he did was wrong and that he regretted it and that he was sincerely sorry and promised her that if she would come back, he would make certain that it would never happened again. Robbie said, "Right now, I am so confused I don't know what to do."

I am not usually this dogmatic, but I said to Robbie, "I can tell you what to do. Continue to stay at your mother's until your husband has had extensive counseling to deal with this problem. When the counselor assures you that he believes your husband has thoroughly worked through this problem, then the two of you can begin to go for marriage counseling. My guess is that his individual counseling will need to last at least six to nine months. The marriage counseling may last almost as long. To go back without thoroughly dealing with the problem is to almost certainly assure that it will happen again. If your husband sincerely wants to deal with the problem, he will go for the counseling and will also give you and your daughter financial assistance while you are living with your mother. If he is not willing to follow through with his counseling and if he seeks to place the blame on you or to manipulate you into coming back by withholding finances, you will know that there can be no reconciliation until his attitude and behavior changes."

Why was I so dogmatic with Robbie? Because research has overwhelmingly shown that a father who has abused multiple children over a long period of time will not change his behavior simply because he is caught. He may cry, he may express sorrow, he may make promises, but none of these can be taken at face value. His actions will speak louder than his words. If he goes for counseling, then there is hope for healing and reconciliation. If he is not willing to go for counseling, there will be no healing.

The greatest thing that Robbie can do for her husband is to practice tough love, and the greatest thing she can do for her daughters is to let them see her doing it. She and her daughters have their own homework to do. Each of the daughters needs counseling and that counseling should involve the mother because chances are the daughters have resentment toward Robbie for allowing this to happen. She may not have known what was going on, but I can almost guarantee you that in their minds, they feel that she is somewhat responsible. If they will each honestly deal with the situation, there can be healing and the girls can rise above the scars of childhood sexual abuse. Dealing with the issues thoroughly at this stage in their lives is far better than glossing over the problem and hoping that the scars of abuse will not show up in their marriages. Unless there is genuine deep healing, the abuse will most certainly have a detrimental effect upon their future relationships.

I don't know what happened to Robbie, her husband, or her daughters. That was my last contact with them; but I do know that I have seen couples in similar situations find healing. I have seen relationships between daughters and fathers renewed. I have seen mothers and daughters work through their own conflicts related to the husband's sexual abuse, and I have seen husbands and wives genuinely reconcile to each other after such devastating abuses. But I have never seen this happen if the abuser is not willing to deal openly, honestly, and thoroughly with his problem.

The spiritual dimension of healing is very important. The acknowledging of moral boundaries and accepting responsibility for breaking these boundaries form an important part of the healing process. Acknowledging wrongdoing, giving and receiving forgiveness, and finding peace with God also are important in healing such relationships. However, religious teachings must never be used to rush a victim to premature and surface forgiveness, and religious conversion must never be used as a quick solution to an abuser's problem. Conversion sets in motion positive changes, but we must not short-circuit the process by assuming that such conversion solves all problems immediately. Religious conversion can chart the course for healing, but we still have to make the journey a day at a time.

For those who have experienced sexual abuse and for those who live with spouses who have, it is my sincere desire that this chapter may serve as the spark to get you started on the road toward healing. Your situation will not exactly parallel the three that we have examined in this chapter, but I trust you will see some common threads that run through all sexual abuse victims and their subsequent marriages. Time alone does not heal the results of sexual abuse. Breaking the barriers of denial, guilt, shame, anger, and fear must precede healing.

All of this begins with a single step. Someone must reach out for help. Usually, it will be the spouse of the abused victim. You can be the positive change agent in your marriage that eventually gets your spouse the help he or she needs in order to find inner healing and, in time, marital healing.

NOTE

1. Cynthia Kubetin and James Mallory, M.D., *Beyond the Darkness: Healing for Victims of Sexual Abuse* (Dallas: Word, 1992).

THE UNFAITHFUL SPOUSE

"I plight thee my troth" was the old English way of saying it. Most modern ceremonies say "I pledge you my faithfulness." At the marriage altar, sexual faithfulness to each other is among the vows we take. Examine most contemporary and historical marriage ceremonies and you will find the idea of sexual faithfulness repeated more than once. When couples come to the marriage altar, they understand that they are committing themselves to be sexually involved with each other and that this means that they will not be sexually involved with anyone else as long as they are married to each other.

Who of us would honestly say "If my spouse desires to have sexual relationships with someone else, it is perfectly fine with me?" Such statements usually are made only by those whose marriage has already died and/or someone who is already involved with someone else and is subconsciously trying to find a way to end the marriage.

Yes, we care about sexual fidelity in marriage. It is not simply a moral or religious concern, although most religions do call for sexual fidelity in marriage. Our concern for sexual faithfulness in marriage is rooted in our humanity. It has to do with integrity and character. It is tied to our emotional need for love. It grows out of a person's desire for an exclusive relationship with someone who will not only value her above all others but also someone to whom she can be fully and totally committed. It is this inner sense of commitment that gives stability to marriage. Sexual infidelity destroys this security and leaves in its wake fear, doubt, distrust, and a sense of betrayal.

Perhaps nothing is more painful to an individual and more destructive to a marriage than discovering that your spouse has been sexually unfaithful to you. Infidelity strikes at the heart of marital unity. We now consider the kinds and causes of sexual unfaithfulness, and loving solutions to restore a marriage broken by such infidelity.

There are different kinds and levels of sexual involvement outside of marriage. The so-called "one-night stand" is the brief, spur-of-the-moment sexual liaison, which is essentially sex without relationship. The long-term affair, on the other hand, begins with an emotional involvement that leads eventually to sexual involvement. Another form of involvement has the spouse finding multiple sexual partners outside the marriage. There are also those who have homosexual or lesbian relationships outside the marriage. Though each of these is somewhat different, they all are devastating to marital intimacy.

SWIRLING EMOTIONS

Before the infidelity is discovered by the spouse, it has a slowly deteriorating effect upon the marriage. After the infidelity is discovered, it stimulates a whirlwind of emotions and reactions on the part of the spouse. It is not information that can simply be accepted on the level of hearing a weather report. It is more like hearing the solemn words of the physician who announces that you or your spouse has some dreaded disease. Denial may be our immediate emotional response, but such denial is typically short lived. The facts are blaring their message so loudly that you cannot ignore them.

If you discover that your spouse has been sexually unfaithful or if he/she reveals such information to you, you will likely experience a cascade of various emotions. Hurt, anger, bitterness, the sense of being betrayed, shame, and perhaps some measure of guilt may all rush to the surface.

Raphael was feeling all of these. Raphael, the bronzed Adonis we met in chapter 1, easily caught women's glances, yet remained devoted to his wife, Joanna. The early years of their marriage had been exciting for both of them, but more recently he felt a growing distance developing in their fifteen-year marriage. He had tried to discuss his feelings with Joanna but she didn't want to talk about it until one day, when she finally let the words rush out: She was involved with a man at work, and they had been lovers for the past two years.

Joanna said that she was sorry and didn't want to hurt him—that was why she hadn't told him before. And while the other man had now left the state and declared the relationship finished, Raphael's wife felt heartbroken; she was still emotionally bonded to him. At times, she felt extremely guilty for what she had done. Raphael had been a good husband. At other times, she knew that she would do it again given the same circumstances. Even now, if her lover called, she would probably get on the first plane to New York.

Raphael was not totally surprised by Joanna's confession. He knew that things had not been right between them for some time. Still, he felt crushed at the thought of Joanna being in the arms of another man. He felt anger toward the other man and pity for Joanna that she had allowed herself to be pulled into such a relationship. He loved Joanna and hoped that they could rebuild their marriage, but he was plagued by the reality that this was not the first time that she had been involved with someone else. Early in their marriage, she had developed an emotional attachment to a man she met playing tennis. She had not gotten sexually involved at that time. At least, she had not shared that with Raphael. But he wondered. He also wondered if there had been other relationships along the way.

The question that plagued him most was: "Will it happen again?" The disappointment, hurt, anger, and worry were over-

whelming at times. He had fleeting thoughts of suicide and linger-
ing thoughts of killing the other man. He loved Joanna in spite of
all that had happened, but he did not know if he could really trust
her again.

Three years after I first met Raphael, I had an extended conversation in which he shared with me what had happened after
Joanna revealed her unfaithfulness to him. What he shared is a
rather classic example of a man who followed the principles of reality living in responding to his wife's sexual unfaithfulness. In the rest
of this chapter, I want to share with you Raphael's story and clarify
the value of handling this crisis in a responsible manner.

RIGHT RESPONSES:
1. REJECT THE MYTHS

First, let me remind you of the four myths that must be rejected if one is to practice reality living.

Myth Number One: My state of mind is determined by my environment.

Myth Number Two: People cannot change.

Myth Number Three: When you are in a bad marriage, there are
only two options: resign yourself to a life of misery or get out of the
marriage.

Myth Number Four: Some situations are hopeless—and my situation is one of these.

Raphael had to wrestle with each of these myths. Any one of
them could have deterred him from taking positive action.
Immediately following Joanna's disclosure, Raphael's most intense
emotion was hurt and disappointment. He wept for a full thirty
minutes after she finished her revelation. He said nothing; he was
too overwhelmed with grief. Then there was the surge of anger,
first toward the other man and later toward Joanna. Then followed
depression: that sense of hopelessness; that nothing could be done
to truly repair the damage, that their marriage was forever lost.

All of these emotions and others rolled in and out of Raphael's
life over the first week. He took no strong action, he made no angry
speeches to Joanna; he found himself withdrawing from her, over-
sleeping in the mornings, and by the end of the first week, decided

172

to take a day off from work and spend some time alone.

It was during this day that Raphael realized that he had an option: He could cave into his emotions and become an angry, bitter, depressed man for the rest of his life; or, despite the painful feelings, he could choose to have a positive attitude and work to make a better future with or without Joanna. He didn't know what direction Joanna would go ultimately, but he knew in his heart that he owed it to himself, his parents, and his friends to think the best and to work toward positive goals.

Over the next couple of weeks, he wrestled with myths number two, three, and four. *People cannot change,* he thought. *If Joanna has been emotionally involved with two men, sexually involved with at least one in our fifteen years of marriage, what assurance do I have that the whole thing would not be repeated three years from now? After all, behavior patterns are hard to change, especially when they involve emotions and the sexual areas of life.* He wondered if he had been deficient somehow in his efforts to be a good husband and had pushed Joanna to become involved with someone else, and, if so, if he could change. He knew that he could not resign himself to a life of misery if Joanna's affairs continued in the future. It was simply not something he was willing to live with.

He thought long and hard about the option of divorce, one option promoted by Myth Number Three. In some ways, he found the idea appealing. If she liked another man, then let her have another man; he would walk his own way. He would build his own happiness, and she would one day regret that she had walked away from him. But he also knew that though divorce would let him walk away from a problem, ultimately it would create other problems. He knew that such action would affect not only him and Joanna but his parents, her parents, and all the extended family who had looked up to them as an ideal couple.

Myth Number Four pounded hard upon his mind: Some situations are hopeless. *Am I batting my head against the wall? Will things ever be different? If they won't, then wouldn't it be better to get out now rather than wasting years following an impossible dream?* All of these myths tugged tenaciously at the coattail of his mind, but at the end of two or three weeks he said no to all of them. He knew others who had fought for their marriage and succeeded. People do change, and perhaps Joanna and he could both make the necessary changes to effect a good marriage. Divorce was not an acceptable option; at least not without making every effort at reconciliation. Why give up now? If it came to divorce, why not make that the last option rather than the first? Maybe Joanna's situation was hopeless, but in his heart he really didn't believe that. Having wrestled with the myths and won, he was now ready to apply the principles of reality living.

2. ACCEPT THE PRINCIPLES OF REALITY LIVING

Let's summarize the principles of reality living: 1. I am responsible for my own attitude. 2. Attitudes affect actions. 3. I cannot change others but I can influence others. 4. My actions are not controlled by my emotions. 5. Admitting my imperfections does not mean that I am a failure. 6. Love is the most powerful weapon for good in the world.

Raphael recognized that he was responsible for his own attitude. Though Joanna's actions had stimulated strong emotions inside of him, he chose to respond to those emotions in a constructive manner. He knew that he could focus on the negative or the positive. He could grovel in his own hurt and anger and eventually become a bitter man, or he could acknowledge his hurt and anger and choose to work his way through these, looking for answers rather than surrendering to their devastating blows. With his positive attitude, he was now ready to take constructive action.

He asked a friend for the name of the counselor who had helped him when he was having a rough time in his marriage. The next day, Raphael called the counselor and made an appointment. He decided to ask Joanna if she wanted to go with him and she agreed. Their appointment with the counselor was exactly six weeks to the day after Joanna had made her revelation about her involvement with the man at work. Joanna had lived in a somewhat depressed state during this time, taking some medication she received from the doctor to get sleep at night. She was generally confused about her feelings and wasn't sure she had the energy to see a counselor, but she agreed to go. Thus began the long and detailed process of finding healing from the fallout of sexual unfaithfulness and rebuilding their marriage.

One of the insights that Raphael gained in counseling was that he could not change Joanna but that his behavior did influence her emotions, which, of course, is reality number three. Nothing he could do would guarantee that Joanna would never be unfaithful again. But he also learned that if they could build an intimate marriage where each of them met the other's emotional need for companionship, it would be the greatest aid against future unfaithfulness.

With the counselor, Raphael and Joanna began to excavate their own needs in a marital relationship and to examine the manner in which these needs had or had not been met in the past. They recognized that each of their needs was unique and if they were to build an intimate marriage, they must both come to understand the other, respect their individual differences, and make genuine efforts at seeking to meet each other's needs.

3. Don't Let the Emotions Take Charge

At times one may want to end the counseling sessions; that's how Raphael felt. He thought the counselor and Joanna were putting undue blame on him for her sexual unfaithfulness, implying that if he had met her needs, she would not have become involved with another man. A part of him wanted to stop the counseling.

When he shared his thinking with the counselor and Joanna, the counselor assured him that it was all right to have those thoughts and feelings.

"Those are typical emotional responses when a couple begins to deal realistically with their marriage. You can leave the counseling process any time you want," he assured Raphael, but the counselor also affirmed the fourth principle of reality living—that our actions need not be controlled by our emotions, that we can acknowledge our emotions and the direction in which they are pushing us but then choose to walk in an opposite direction, believing the overall benefit of doing so will be positive. Raphael stayed in counseling, and the process of reconciliation went forward.

One of the most difficult parts of the counseling for Raphael was admitting that he had not been as successful in meeting

Joanna's emotional needs as he had assumed through the years. He discovered, for example, that Joanna had felt left out of the decision-making process because he often made decisions without discussing them with her. Raphael was a strong, confident, insightful businessman. He made decisions daily in the business and prided himself on being a good decision-maker. When it came to decision-making in the marriage, he had always considered Joanna's needs and made his decisions with her in mind. In fact, she had been pleased with most of his decisions, but she still felt isolated and left out of the process. She viewed him more as a father who was making benevolent decisions for his children. She saw herself as a child rather than a partner whose ideas and feelings were welcomed at the discussion table.

This perception of him as a father rather than a partner had been a part of what had motivated her to look elsewhere for intimacy. Understanding and admitting these emotional dynamics was extremely painful for Raphael. He was helped by principle number five: Admitting my imperfections does not mean that I am a failure. The counselor helped Raphael understand that his intentions had been positive; his method of decision-making had been loving and altruistic toward Joanna; but it had not served her emotional need for companionship. Admitting this did not mean that he had been a failure; it simply meant that there was a better way to make decisions, and this involved communication with Joanna. With the counselor, the husband and wife negotiated the changes they would make in the decision-making process.

There were several other discoveries made in the counseling process that helped Raphael understand that changes needed to be made in the way in which he related to Joanna. Together, they learned how to tell each other their feelings, thoughts, and desires without condemning the other person. They learned how to make requests rather than demands. They learned the joy of making changes in order to meet each other's needs. In short, they did the hard work of building an intimate marriage relationship.

Like most couples who choose counseling, this couple met the counselor in both individual and joint sessions. In the individual sessions, we often work through personal attitudes and emotions.

The counselor helped Joanna deal with the deep emotions she still felt for the other man. She came to understand that these emotions would not subside overnight; that the memories of their times together would often flash in her mind and the desire for the intimacy which they shared would often dominate her thinking. Assured by the counselor that her actions did not have to follow these emotions and desires, Joanna continued to work on rebuilding her relationship with Raphael. She chose to say "no thank you" to the two or three phone calls she received from New York. She knew in her heart that to pursue that relationship was a dead-end street. She knew that Raphael had been faithful to her and that he loved her; otherwise, he would not be willing to forgive her of her indiscretions. Over a period of about a year, her feelings of intimacy toward Raphael grew, and her feelings and memories of the other man diminished. She knew that she was on the road toward healing.

FORGIVE—AND ASK FORGIVENESS

One of the most difficult times for Joanna came after about nine months of counseling when she began to experience intensely Raphael's love and to understand how deeply she had hurt him. In the early part of counseling, she had focused on Raphael's failures and had tried to shift the blame of her unfaithfulness. But by now she knew that it was a two-way street and that she must take responsibility for her own actions. Her guilt weighed heavily upon her, and she realized that she had never sincerely and deeply asked Raphael for forgiveness.

Early in the process of recovery, she had intellectually acknowledged that what she did was wrong and she had asked for Raphael's forgiveness. But this time she needed his forgiveness on a much deeper level. Now she was keenly aware of her own guilt; now she understood the gift of forgiveness that Raphael had offered her. She said the words again: "Please forgive me for all the pain I have caused you." Raphael responded, "I do."

With deep emotion and many tears, they embraced. And they both knew that from that point, healing from the past was assured. Now her sexual unfaithfulness would become only a scar, not an open wound.

In the early stages of recovery, one of Raphael's deep struggles was living with the awareness that his wife still had strong emotional feelings for another man with whom she had been sexually active. These realities often rained on his parade. He wanted so hard to let the past go but it was so difficult when he knew that she still had thoughts and feelings for the other man. The counselor assured him that living with this reality was a part of the process of recovery, that if she denied that she had these feelings, they would not be building an authentic relationship. The important thing was that she was choosing him over the other man. She was not allowing her emotions to control her actions and that Raphael could give thanks for her choices if not for her feelings.

After their night of forgiveness, Raphael knew that his long struggle was over, that Joanna now understood his pain and genuinely regretted all that she had put him through. He knew now that her feelings were for him and that their marriage was going to make it.

For marital healing after unfaithfulness, forgiveness is essential. It involves two key elements: confession and asking for forgiveness on the part of the erring spouse, and genuine forgiveness on the part of the offended. Forgiveness is a promise: "I will no longer hold that against you." Such forgiveness takes place on different emotional levels; thus, Joanna desired to repeat the forgiving process nine months into the counseling session. When we forgive, we must include not only the sexual unfaithfulness, but other failures that come to light as we take an honest look at our marriage relationship.

For Raphael and Joanna, the counseling continued for several months, but now with an air of confidence rather than the palling uncertainty of the early months of recovery. Raphael and Joanna each could now give themselves to the other more fully because trust had been reborn and commitment expressed. Anger, guilt, fear, and anxiety had all been processed. They had demonstrated to each other reality principle number six: love is the most powerful weapon for good in the world. When we choose the loving actions of confessing failures, extending forgiveness, and genuinely seeking to meet the needs of each other, marital intimacy becomes reality.

The illusive dream is no longer illusive or a dream.

WRONG RESPONSES

Having reflected upon Raphael and Joanna's journey to recovery after sexual unfaithfulness, I now want to look at some of the common pitfalls that hinder couples in their journey on the road of reality living. As noted earlier, discovering sexual unfaithfulness on the part of your spouse is like the exploding of a bombshell in your marriage. Things cannot go on as normal. Emotions must now be processed, and decisions must now be made. How we respond to these emotions and decisions will move us toward restoration or divorce.

Hurt and anger are two of the most common emotions upon learning of a spouse's unfaithfulness. These are deep and powerful emotions. They can push us to homicide or abandonment. In anger, we can pull the trigger and kill the guilty party or we can turn and walk out the door and never return. One alternative leads to death, the other to divorce, but neither deals with the issues that give rise to the unfaithfulness. And both create another whole set of problems with which we must now deal.

Hurt and anger are healthy emotions. They reveal that you are human and that you care about your marriage relationship. They indicate that you see yourself as a valuable person who has been wronged. They reveal your concern for rightness and fairness. These emotions need to be processed in a positive way.

Initially, crying, weeping, and sobbing are healthy responses to the emotions of hurt and anger. However, the body is limited in how long it can sustain such agony; thus, sessions of weeping must be interspersed with periods of calm.

Expressing verbally your hurt and anger to the unfaithful spouse is a healthy way of processing anger. It is better if you can express your anger with "I" statements rather than "you" statements, which can sound accusing and provoke a defensive or aggressive response. Here are some examples of "I" statements: "I feel betrayed . . . I feel hurt . . . I feel used; I feel taken advantage of . . . I feel that you don't love me; I feel that you could never have loved me . . . I feel unclean . . . I feel like I don't ever want to touch you again."[1]

All of these statements reveal your thoughts and feelings to your spouse. They are honest, they are not cloaked; they are communicating to your spouse the deep hurt, pain, and anger which you feel. Any recovery requires that your spouse hear and understand the depth of your hurt and anger.

On the other hand, "you" statements tend not only to condemn but to incite further negative reaction from your spouse. If, for example, you use the following statements expressing the same sentiments, they tend to incite battle rather than understanding. "You betrayed me . . . you hurt me . . . you took advantage of me . . .you don't love me; you could never have loved me." Such statements place blame and incite negative reactions, while "I" statements simply reveal your emotions.

Another way of processing your anger and hurt is to share it with a trusted friend, minister, or counselor. Verbalizing the hurt and anger to another person is a healthy way of working through the anger to a positive resolution.

On the other hand, there are many negative responses to anger that complicate the problem. If in your anger you start throwing glasses and dishes, you may not only physically hurt your spouse and be liable for physical abuse, but you may destroy some of your prized possessions. If this is done in the presence of children, you also give them a visual image of a mother or father out of control. This image is extremely difficult for children to process. Such angry outbursts accompanied by physical threats or actions may land you in jail and further compound your problems. They also alleviate some of the guilt of your spouse; now he can blame you rather than himself because your behavior has demonstrated that you are an unreasonable, uncontrolled person. Removing his guilt or giving him the opportunity to shift the guilt to you is not a part of the recovery process; it pushes him further toward divorce.

Retaliation is another common but very negative response to an unfaithful spouse. Such retaliation may involve going out and having an affair yourself to show her what it feels like to be betrayed. Other vengeful tactics are to go to her place of work and cause a scene with angry shouting and yelling. If the unfaithful spouse moves out of the house and continues to see the new partner, a vengeful response would be to drive by their dwelling, throw bricks through a window, call their number and either be silent or sound off, or let the air out of the tires of their cars; or, as in one case I remember, remove the battery from the car. These tactics are juvenile and detrimental as well as being unlawful.

Any effort at revenge is doomed to failure. Returning wrong for wrong simply makes the other person feel less guilty and tends to stimulate within him the desire to return fire for fire. Thus the problem escalates rather than finding resolution.

THE NEED FOR COUNSELING

There are many questions that must be answered and many decisions that must be made after the revelation that a spouse has been sexually unfaithful. These questions and decisions are best made with the help of a professional counselor or a trusted friend who can help both of you think clearly about the best steps to take. Sometimes the erring spouse will not be willing to go for counseling. Then go alone. Start the process. If she is not willing to deal with the situation, you must deal with your own emotions and your own decisions. You are far more likely to make wise decisions if you get the help of someone who is not emotionally involved in the situation.

If you go for counseling, your spouse may eventually join you, even if he is reluctant to do so in the beginning. If he never joins you, you can walk the road of reality living and whether or not the marriage is restored, you can live a better life in the future than you have lived in the past.

In my opinion, restoration is the goal toward which one should work when a spouse has been unfaithful. But obviously, this is not always possible. The spouse may be unwilling to break off the sexual liaison, or the partner may promise to break it off and in fact continue. He or she may actually break it but later begin another relationship. We cannot make someone deal with his or her problems but we can deal with our own problems. The challenge of reality living is to take responsibility for our own thoughts and actions and seek to do the most constructive thing in each of life's difficult situations. This is the best approach for our own mental and spiritual health. It has the added possibility of stimulating positive change in the life of the spouse.

NOTE

1. Depending on one's personality, an offended spouse may feel many different responses. It is perfectly acceptable to say any of the following to convey your frustration or anger: "I feel like I am going to suffocate . . . I feel like I wish I could die . . . I feel like I could kill that other person . . . I feel like I could kill you. . .I am so confused; I don't understand . . . I thought we had a good marriage . . . I feel like I must have failed you . . . I feel like I want you to leave; I feel like I want to get out of here."

THE ALCOHOLIC/ DRUG-ABUSING SPOUSE

*A*lcoholism is a family problem. The drinking and subsequent behavior of the alcoholic harms not only the life of the alcoholic but the lives of all who interact with him or her. Numerous volumes have been written on the adverse effects of parental alcoholism upon children. In this chapter, we focus our attention on what alcoholism does to a marriage.

In truth, few things damage marital intimacy more than alcoholism. In fact, research has shown that a marriage in which one partner is a drug or alcohol abuser has a one-in-ten chance of survival.[1] With an estimated twelve million alcoholics in the United States, we are dealing with a problem of colossal magnitude.

Drug abuse is equally damaging to marital intimacy. Why are these two substances, alcohol and drugs, so destructive to the marital relationship? The answer lies in the behavior that grows out of substance abuse. The substance abuser lives in an egocentric world. In a general sense that is true of all of us, but it is profoundly true of the substance abuser. The abuser of alcohol or drugs is inwardly directed and absorbed with his own pain or pleasure, and thus has a very self-centered life. This self-centeredness impairs his normal day-to-day living and his personal relationships. The pattern of behavior brings destructive traits to the marital relationship.

What are these destructive traits? The most serious is dishonesty. In her effort to hide her addiction, the abuser becomes a master of deceit. Such deceit is the antithesis of intimacy. It builds walls between marital partners. Other aspects of the alcoholic behavior pattern include an unwillingness to face conflict, emotional distance from the marriage partner, lack of empathy, and what appears to be a disinterest in the spouse. Her addiction makes her insensitive to the feelings of those who care for her. The addict's highest priority in life is using the addicting substance. She will stop at nothing to feed the addiction. Even though she knows that her use of drugs or alcohol causes her spouse deep pain, she continues the practice and is willing to let the spouse suffer.

While under the influence, addicts often engage in behavior that ultimately destroys the marriage. Acts of sexual infidelity are characteristic of alcoholics. The fact that he was drunk at the time is little consolation to a grief-stricken wife. Physical and emotional neglect and abuse are also characteristic of those under the influence. Even when he is not abusive, his talk and behavior may evoke disgust, pity, and anger in the heart of the spouse. Life with a substance abuser makes marital intimacy seem impossible.

FEELINGS OF HOPELESSNESS

Barbara, whom we met in chapter 1, knew the sense of hopelessness that comes from living with an alcoholic husband. She shared with me that her husband, Dan, drank some before they got married, but after marriage his drinking became a bigger part of his life. For the past ten years, his alcoholism had been tearing at their marriage. It led to verbal abuse and loss of jobs. After each lost job, Dan would go on a drinking binge, followed by the drying-out period and then a new job search. A new job led to new hope, but the drinking would resume, and the cycle began anew.

Barbara could tell where they were in the cycle. She also knew what was coming next. She really did not want a divorce. But things had only gotten worse, despite her deep religious faith and talks with Dan about the problem. "I'm to the point that I don't know what to do now. I find my love feelings for him dying and being replaced by pity and anger. I want to respect him. I want to love him. I want to help him, but I don't know how," she said. Ten years seemed like an eternity and Barbara was thinking seriously of the one thing she never wanted—divorce.

BEING AN "ENABLER"

In talking further with Barbara, I found that in many ways she was the classic enabler. Unwittingly, she had helped Dan continue his addictive lifestyle. Her father was an alcoholic, which is often the case of wives who find themselves married to alcoholics. In childhood, she had learned the skills of overlooking disruptive behavior, trying to keep peace in the family, excusing her father's behavior, and longing for the day when things would be different. Barbara now used these unconscious skills to foster Dan's alcoholism.

The enabler feels compelled to try at all costs to decrease the chaos which the alcohol or drug use produces. In so doing, he or she only perpetuates the addiction. Without an enabler, it would be difficult for the user to continue the habit. The enabler often feels anger, but this is hidden by a genuine concern for the other person. The enabler is patient and unselfish and often overprotects and tries to rescue the substance abuser. The payoff is a shallow peace that cannot lead to marital intimacy.

I knew that if Barbara were to ever become a positive change agent in her marriage, she would have to change her thinking and her behavior. She would have to learn to give up the responsibility of her husband's behavior and accept responsibility for her own behavior. She would have to let Dan suffer the consequences of his addictive lifestyle. For many spouses of substance abusers, this fundamental change of behavior must take place. The spouse must recognize that the only thing that ultimately motivates a drug user to make the decision to get off drugs and seek treatment is suffering the consequences of his lifestyle. Then the abuser may realize that to continue in that lifestyle is to lose everything that is important to him. This realization most often comes as the result of a crisis.

This may be the loss of a job, severe illness, being arrested, the separation of a spouse, or the rejection of family and friends. It is only when the addict comes to despise his own lifestyle that he/she will be motivated to seek treatment.

Barbara had come to me for marital counseling, but I knew that such counseling would be fruitless unless the addiction problem was addressed. Continuing alcoholism and drug abuse sabotage all such efforts. My first suggestion was that Barbara begin attending the local Al–Anon chapter. Al–Anon is a national organization that provides information and support to family members of substance abusers. It offers them the practical insights and the emotional support to become positive change agents. They come to realize that though they cannot control the addicted behavior of their loved one, they can influence him.[2]

Alcoholism and other addictions tend to isolate families. Shame, uncertainty, and fear of the unknown often paralyze the spouse into inactivity. What Barbara learned at Al–Anon was that she was not alone. Millions of men and women are married to alcoholics who have experienced a similar history in their own marriages. Their lives also have become unmanageable. But she also found hope. The first step was to accept responsibility for her own actions. The second step was to let Dan accept responsibility for his actions. She learned that she did not cause Dan's drinking, she could not control it, nor could she cure it. She learned that trying to be loving and supportive of the drug addict in a caretaking manner only makes the situation worse. She learned that drug addiction causes one to regress emotionally to become extremely immature, and that alcoholics learn how to manipulate, con, and lie in order to be successful addicts. Their stories and excuses sound so plausible that the spouse is inclined to believe them.

Barbara learned how to admit the truth that Dan had used her all these years to continue his addictive behavior. It was now time for her to refuse to be his pawn and to become a strong pillar of tough love. She learned how to genuinely love him by refusing to pick up the pieces, to make excuses, or to rescue him from the consequences of his behavior.

She remembers well the difficulty of letting him stay in the local jail in spite of his pleadings for her to get him out. She called a friend from Al–Anon. They prayed and cried together on the telephone. The thought of Dan spending the night in jail was extremely painful for Barbara, but she knew that her refusal to bail him out was her strongest expression of love at the moment.

Tough Love in Action

Over the next year, she watched Dan lose his job, knowing that if she had jumped in and helped like she used to, she could have saved his job. But she realized that there was something more important than saving Dan's job; namely, helping Dan accept responsibility for his own behavior.

After Dan lost his job, he went on another drinking binge. This is when Barbara took the two children and moved in with her mother. This was the last straw for Dan.

He came begging and pleading for Barbara to return. He promised that he would never drink again, that he had learned his lesson. With the support of her friends at Al–Anon, Barbara was able to say no to Dan's tears. She would not return until he entered a treatment program and even then, she would not return until they had marriage counseling. There would be no more fast fixes. Unless Dan would deal with his alcoholism and unless he were willing to work with her on learning how to build a good marriage, she would never return.

Dan came back the next night and begged for Barbara's return. He would go to treatment if she would just return. Barbara recognized this as a further attempt to manipulate her. Her response was a kind, firm no.

"I love you too much to return to you now," she told him. "I will not short-circuit the process. If I return, it will be after you have dealt with your alcoholism and after we have dealt with our marital problems." She told him of a treatment program in a nearby city and assured him that she would work with him on getting into the program, that in fact, she and the children would come on occasion for counseling sessions with him at the treatment center's request.

"Dan, we have a serious problem," she continued. "It is not going to go away by itself. We all need help. This is your chance to decide if you want your marriage and family or if you want to live with alcohol for the rest of your life."

Within three days, Dan was in the treatment center, and for the next three months, Dan entered a whole new world; a world of reality; a world where people accepted responsibility for their own actions and emotions; a world where people learned to understand themselves and the value of relating to others. He learned about alcoholism, but he learned more about himself. For the first time in his life, Dan began to realize that life in the real world could be much more satisfying than life in the delusional world of alcohol.

At the end of the ninety-day treatment program (in which Barbara and the children also participated under the direction of their counselor), Dan was released with the full understanding that he and Barbara would not be living together until they had received sufficient marriage counseling to heal the emotional hurts of the past ten years and to build new patterns of relating to each other in marriage. This time, Dan was not begging for Barbara to return. He was living in the real world and knew that he had deeply hurt Barbara with his self-centered, destructive behavior over the past ten years and that he had to allow time for her healing. He also recognized that he had a great deal to learn about how to relate to his wife and his children.

We began extensive marriage and family counseling, which nine months later resulted in Barbara and the children moving back home. Dan continued to attend Alcoholics Anonymous (AA) meetings once a week during the time of our marriage counseling. Barbara likewise saw her need for personal growth and continued her weekly meetings with her friends in Al–Anon. Dan had only one brief relapse during the nine months. He was at a business meeting and thought that he could have a drink socially without getting drunk. One drink led to two and before the evening was over, Dan had to be taken home in a taxi. The next week he went to AA meetings each day and shared his relapse with his AA support group. He also shared this information with Barbara and later with me in our counseling session. This openness was far different from Dan's previous style of denial and lying. Barbara and Dan both had a high level of confidence that their marriage would be vastly different from the past ten years. I continued to see them monthly for the first six months after they moved back together and semi-annually for two years after that.

As of this writing, it's been five years since I last counseled with Barbara and Dan, but every Christmas I've received a card and a brief note recounting some of the events of the year. Always they express their gratitude.

Barbara and Dan's story is a success case. (There is success but never a cure. An alcoholic is only one drink away from the obsession.) Unfortunately, most spouses married to substance abusers end up divorcing them. They have tried sensible conversation, angry lectures, silent withdrawal, crying, pleading, trying to save face, making excuses, picking up the pieces, and hoping against hope that their spouse will change.

The fact is that most addicts do not change—until their personal pain becomes so intense that it is unbearable. This pain may come from any of the natural consequences of their addiction such as loss of job, physical illness, rejection of friends. But the deepest pain that an addict can experience is the thought of losing a spouse or some other deeply significant person in his life. That is what motivated Dan to seek treatment and that is what motivates most addicts to seek treatment. The thought of losing the one person who means the most to them in the whole world is enough pain to motivate many addicts to reach out for help.

This means that the spouse or other significant person must be strong enough not to cave in to the initial manipulation of the alcoholic, but must stand kindly but firmly for the necessary long-term treatment, which includes follow-up meetings with AA or another appropriate support group. Most spouses and significant others will not be strong enough to take this tough love approach without the guidance and support of a group like Al–Anon. After all, most of these people have a ten- or fifteen-year record of being an enabler. These patterns do not change easily. Even when the spouse begins to practice tough love, well-meaning friends and family may accuse him/her of abandoning the alcoholic. Thus, the first positive step that any family member of an alcoholic can take is to become a part of an educational support group such as Al–Anon.

AVAILABLE PROGRAMS FOR SUBSTANCE ABUSERS

Another significant step in the process of being a positive change agent is to discover the treatment center options available so that when the time comes that your spouse is willing to go for treatment, you will be ready to suggest a treatment center. There are three basic formats for treating drug abusers. One is *outpatient therapy*. The outpatient program typically provides a time for detoxification if needed, weekly meetings, individual and group counseling, peer counseling, and frequent urine drug screening. Peer counseling and urine screening are extremely important. The addict cannot con other addicts. Confrontation by their peers is strong confrontation. Knowing that one is going to be tested for drugs is a strong deterrent and motivates the drug user to say no to temptation. Outpatient programs are less expensive and less disruptive to one's work and family relationships. They work best with people who are in good health and have a strong desire to become drug free.

Inpatient treatment is a more intensive program. It usually involves detoxification, educational training, group and individual therapy, family involvement, and sometimes occupational and recreational therapy. Such a program may last six weeks to three months and at the end introduces the patient to Alcoholics Anonymous or some other follow-up group. Inpatient treatment has the advantage of being intensive and removes the drug user from both the drug and the drug-using environment. Those who have been addicted for a long period of time, are in poor health, or whose living environment encourages drug use usually need an inpatient program.

A third approach is *residential programs*. These programs offer long-term treatment in a controlled environment where the recovering drug user can learn how to live without drugs. Residential programs usually run from six months to a year. They utilize a very structured program, keeping the patient constructively busy and away from drugs and drug-using friends. The residential program usually offers dormitory-style living, daily responsibilities in caring for the facility, family-style meals, and a fairly disciplined environment. Usually educational and vocational training are included, along with group activities. Typically counseling focuses not only on treating drug abuse but on dealing with any underlying emotional/relational problems. Residential programs are more commonly used with adolescents or young adults than with older adults.

Certain drug treatment programs have had more success than others—success being defined as drug-free living accompanied by responsible living and positive growing relationships after the treatment. The most successful treatment programs are characterized by the following elements: (1) a commitment to a drug-free environment and a goal of total abstinence, (2) competent medical and nursing care, (3) a strong emphasis on one's personal spiritual life, (4) educational sessions that provide understanding of the effects of drugs, (5) both group and individual therapy sessions, (6) involvement of the larger family (spouse, children, or others) in the treatment process, and (7) a strong commitment to getting the patient into a support group after the initial treatment program.

Information on available treatment centers may be secured through your Al–Anon support group, a local counselor or minister, your local mental health clinic, or by talking with friends. It is always advisable to learn as much about a treatment program as possible early in the process so that when your spouse is ready for treatment, you will be ready with a viable suggestion. Most treatment programs welcome visits and are happy to discuss with family members their methods and costs of treatments. Costs vary greatly among treatment programs. Most health insurance programs have provision for addiction treatment. All of these details should be known and understood long before the spouse is willing to go for treatment.

The most common mistake of an individual married to a substance abuser is to simply hope that the situation will take care of itself, that the abuser will wake up one morning and decide to stop her addictive behavior. The reality is that this almost never happens. When one is truly addicted, it is not a matter of simply deciding to get off the drug. At this point, the body has a physical addiction to the drug and will drive the addict incessantly to meet that need. Once addicted, the substance abuser will need outside help to break the destructive habit.

The role of the spouse who would be a positive change agent is to let the abuser experience the results of his/her own abuse. The sooner the abuser comes to the end of the rope, the sooner he will reach out for help. It often takes years for the disease of alcoholism to disable the addict physically to the point that non-family members are aware there is a problem. Long before that, the spouse knows and needs to love enough to confront the reality of the disease. The spouse is there to insist that the use of alcohol and its resultant behavior is not acceptable. Things cannot go on as usual. When spouses affirm by their actions that they will no longer make excuses nor get the abuser off the hook, they are doing the good work of tough love. The potential of the spouse deciding to seek treatment is now in place. Without this tough love approach, the potential for change is almost nil.

Finally, don't ignore the important role of the spiritual life both for the abuser and the caring spouse in overcoming the addiction. Research has made it abundantly clear that the most successful treatment programs are those programs which point the individual to the help and power of God. In fact, the first two steps of the Alcoholic Anonymous Twelve Step program recognize that we are helpless to change without God,[3] and many alcoholics who had no spiritual reference points earlier find themselves seeking and benefiting from their call for divine help. There is nothing wrong or sissy about that. The addict is helpless to change himself but with the help of God, no addict is hopeless.

As for the spouse who is seeking to be a positive change agent, the pain of observing an addicted mate often seems overwhelming. Your sense of isolation from friends and family may cause you to feel alone. You too need the help of God and God's representatives—fellow humans who love, care, and are knowledgeable about how to relate redemptively to those who are addicted. The most important step you can take is to pray for God's guidance and then call a friend, pastor, counselor, or the local Al–Anon group.

With the support of God and others, you can take the road of tough love. It is the only love that will truly help the alcoholic or drug-abusing spouse.

NOTES

1. Stephen Van Cleave, Walter Byrd, and Kathy Revell, *Counseling for Substance Abuse and Addiction* (Dallas: Word, 1987), 90.
2. To find a local chapter of Al–Anon, check the yellow pages in your telephone directory or call the national headquarters at 1-800-344-2666.
3. The first two steps of the Twelve Steps of Alcoholics Anonymous are: 1. We admitted we were powerless over alcohol—that our lives had become unmanageable. 2. Came to believe that a Power greater than ourselves could restore us to sanity.

THE DEPRESSED SPOUSE

*J*ohn, an active businessman in his early forties, was trying to get his business up and running. He could now see the fruit of his hard work beginning to pay off, but sitting in my office, it was obvious that John was not a happy man.

"Dr. Chapman, I've worked hard. I've been under a lot of stress for the last three years. Some people told me that the business would not make it, but I was determined. Now I know that we have turned the corner. The business is on solid ground, and I am certain that it will grow over the next few years. My problem is not with my business; it's with my wife.

"She seems so unhappy and sad almost all of the time. I don't remember the last time I saw her smile. She is so negative and pessimistic about everything. She has been prophesying the demise of the business for the last year and a half. She spends most mornings in bed, and in the afternoons she just sits around the house. She seems to have no ambition. She does get the children a snack when they come home from school, and she talks with them a bit about their day. But every night, I have to bring food home for dinner. She says that she doesn't have the energy to cook. Many nights, she doesn't eat with us. She must have lost forty pounds over the last year. She's up and down all night long; says she can't sleep. This, of course, makes it hard for me to sleep. She worries about everything.

"To be truthful, life is pretty miserable at our house. I feel sorry for the kids, although they get more attention than I do. But I know that they must wonder what is wrong with their mother. She seems so depressed all the time."

With that brief description, John had just given the common symptoms of depression. For the depressed person, the mood will be sad, the thinking negative, and the behavior lifeless. Physically, the depressed person may exhibit loss of appetite, loss of weight, poor or excessive sleep, or loss of sexual drive. These characteristics are often accompanied by general anxiety. The person will express fears, uncertainty, and indecisiveness. Thousands of men and women can identify with John's frustration because they too live with a depressed spouse. Unfortunately, many of them have little understanding of the causes and cures of depression. They simply do not understand why their spouses cannot "snap out of it and get on with life." Lack of understanding often stimulates frustration and a critical spirit. Their words of criticism actually compound the problem.

THREE CATEGORIES OF DEPRESSION

Understanding depression is not a simple matter. There are many types of depression, each with its own specific cause and each producing varying levels of depression. It is beyond the scope of this chapter to give a full treatise on understanding depression, but let me give a brief overview. It is helpful to think of three categories of depression. First, depression may be the *by-product of a physical illness*. For example, when you have a full-blown case of influenza, you don't care what is going on at the office. You want to lie still and sleep as much as possible. You lose all interest in the outside world. You temporarily check out; your mind and emotions have moved into a depressed state. It is nature's way of protecting you from constant anxiety about what you are missing in the real world. Fortunately, the influenza passes and your depressive mood lifts, though you may have noted that it tends to hang on for a day or two after your physical symptoms are gone. It often takes the mind a couple of days to get back to its normal state.

A second kind of depression is often called *situational depression* or *reactive depression*. It is the depression that grows out of a particular painful situation in life. Such depression is a reaction to those painful experiences. Most of these experiences involve a sense of loss. For example, depression often follows the loss of a spouse by death or divorce, the loss of a job, the loss of a child to college, the loss of parents to death, the loss of a friendship, the loss of money. Depression may also arise over the loss of a dream, such as a happy, fulfilling marriage, the loss of the love feelings that you once had for your spouse, or the loss of hope that your marriage will ever be as fulfilling as you once hoped.

A third category is depression rooted in some biochemical disorder, which has put the mind and emotions in a state of disequilibrium. Sometimes this is referred to as *endogenous depression*. The word *endogenous* means "from within the body," and the biological-chemical change inside the body is its source. This is depression as a sort of physical disease.

There are various forms of biological depression. Some are related directly to the brain where something goes wrong with the electrical and neurochemical transmissions. Others are related to disorders of the endocrine system. The glands of the endocrine system (thyroid, parathyroid, thymus, pancreas, pituitary, adrenal, ovaries, and gonads) produce hormones that are released into the blood stream to perform various functions. Lowered or heightened levels of these hormones can produce depression. Also, certain disorders of metabolism can produce depression. The body is constantly assimilating food, breaking it into substances that can be stored and used as energy. When things go wrong in the metabolic system, depression can sometimes result. For example, abnormally low blood sugar levels can produce feelings of emotional instability and depression.

There may well be biological reasons why females are more prone to depression than males. The female reproductive organs are known to create mood swings. Premenstrual syndrome, commonly known as PMS, is the depression at the onset of menstruation; it is a common occurrence. Women in menopause often face bouts of depression. The variation in estrogen levels markedly influences the mood of women.

The good news about biologically caused depression is that it is readily treated with medication. The bad news is that only about one-third of all depressions are biological depressions. The far more common depression is situational depression. Medications are of little or no value in treating situational depressions unless, of course, the situational depression has gone on for a long period of time and has affected the biochemistry of the body. It is true that extended periods of depression, whatever the original cause, may lead to problems in the neurochemical transmission system in the brain. Thus, medication may be a part of a treatment program.

Most all of us from time to time experience brief bouts of situational depression. These are simply our normal responses to the problems of everyday life. Usually we are not overwhelmed by these feelings of depression, nor do we allow them to control our behavior, and in a few days these feelings have passed; the depression was of little consequence in the overall flow of life. At other times, however, depression becomes a serious problem. The term often used of these more serious periods of depression is *clinical depression*. This term is used in many ways, but more commonly it is used to refer to a depression that has lingered for many weeks or perhaps months, and the depression has affected the normal functions of life, such as sleep, appetite, capacity for work, and social relationships. As a clinical depression, the condition needs treatment; it is not likely to go away simply with more time. If treatment is not secured, the depression will tend to deepen, and the person will become more and more withdrawn from the realities of life. It is the task of the treatment specialist to determine the cause of the depression and to suggest a course of treatment.

THE DOCTOR'S ROLE, THE COUNSELOR'S ROLE

Most depressed persons who reach out for help turn first to their medical doctor. However, most medical doctors do not have time to give a thorough analysis to determine the cause of the depression. Thus, physicians often prescribe what is commonly referred to as an antidepressant medication. If the depression happens to have a biological cause, then the medication can be helpful. It usually takes three to four weeks to determine if a given medication is producing positive results. If it does not, the physician often will try another type of medication. It is not uncommon for a doctor to prescribe three or four different types of medication before there is any noticeable change in the patient's depressive state.

However, if the individual's depression does not have a biological cause, the medication will be of little value. Since only about a third of depression has a biological root, it is far more advisable for the depressed person to begin with a trained counselor who has experience in treating those who are depressed. By nature of his/her profession, the counselor has more time to explore the root cause of the depression. If it is in fact a situational depression, then counseling is the best method of treatment. The person must come to process his/her grief over the loss that stimulated the depression or learn to adapt to the situation which caused the depression. This is best done over a period of time with a trained counselor. If the counselor discerns that there may be a biochemical aspect to the person's depression, he/she normally will refer the individual to a psychiatrist, who after evaluation will recommend a particular medication. A combination of medication and counseling is the best treatment for these individuals.

As for depressions that are the by-product of a physical disease such as influenza, cancer, or any other chronic disease, counseling can be helpful for the depression and medical treatment is certainly recommended to treat the disease itself. Usually, there is mutual respect for the value of both the physician and the counselor, each dealing with a different aspect of an individual's problem.

In all depressions, the spiritual aspect of life is an important part of the patient's treatment. Most professionals recognize a connection between the physical, psychological, and spiritual aspects of life. The counselor who is unwilling to explore the area of spiritual renewal is in my opinion overlooking one of the most helpful aspects of treating depression. On the other hand, there is always the danger of religious enthusiasts who see all depression as a spiritual problem and thus heap more guilt upon the depressed person. Such an approach, far from being helpful, actually exacerbates the depression. The healthiest road of treatment involves an honest and in-depth evaluation of all three elements: physical, psychological, and spiritual. Depression is not an incurable disease. Even those who have been depressed for months or sometimes years can find relief with the proper treatment.

As John sat in my office sharing his struggle with his wife Debbie's behavior, it was obvious to me that he had little understanding of these concepts. He knew that Debbie had a problem, and he knew that her problem was causing him great frustration. But he wasn't even sure what Debbie's problem was and he certainly had no idea of how to help her. For a while he had tried to listen to her sympathetically. He had given her his best advice. But he had seen no progress and had become frustrated. Eventually he was giving her angry lectures, with such hurtful comments as, "You are destroying our marriage, and you have no idea how detrimental this is to the children. You need to get hold of yourself."

John arrived at my office in one final, last-ditch effort. He had been thinking of divorce for some time, feeling that he could not live the rest of his life in such a stressful marriage.

I was sympathetic with John's frustration, but I knew in my heart that divorce was not the answer. My first suggestion was to ask John to read a book on depression. Until he gained some understanding of the nature of depression, I knew that he would not be able to be a positive change agent. When he came back the following week, he had read the entire book and said to me, "There is no question about it. Debbie is depressed. She has all the characteristics. I don't know if it is a biological depression or a situational depression, but I know that she is depressed." I could tell that he had read the book thoughtfully.

Now that we both had agreed on the problem, the question was how to get Debbie the help she needed. I asked, "Do you think that Debbie would come in to see me if you told her that you have talked with me about your own frustrations in the marriage and that I had requested that she make an appointment?"

"I don't know," John responded. "She hasn't been out of the house in at least two weeks. I don't know how she would respond if I told her that."

"Would you be willing to try?" I continued. "Simply tell her that you have been to see me and shared with me some of your frustrations in the marriage and that I had requested that she call and make an appointment with my secretary." Then I said to John, "If she doesn't call my secretary in a week, do I have your permission to call her and tell her that I've talked with you and that I would like very much for her to come in and see me? I will tell her that I feel that I cannot help you without talking to her."

"That's fine with me," John said. "I don't have anything to lose at this point."

"One other request," I said to John. "Don't mention the word *depression* to Debbie. Just tell her that you talked with me about your frustrations in the marriage." John agreed. (I didn't want Debbie to get the idea that the two of us had ganged up, diagnosed her problem, and were now out to cure her.)

AN INTERVIEW WITH DEBBIE

The next week came and went without a call from Debbie. The following week I called her and asked that she come in to see me. Four days later, she was in my office, with her clothes hanging loosely on her thin body and her face void of expression. I explained why I had asked her to come to my office: that after John shared with me his own struggles in the marriage, I felt like I could not respond to him unless I found out her perspective on the marriage. I told her I wanted to ask her a few questions and that I wanted her to be honest with me about how she viewed her marriage.

I asked the normal questions regarding how long she had been married, how many children they had, and, on a scale of 0–10, to tell me how healthy she viewed their marriage as being. Her answer to the last question was "2." At least she was in touch with that reality.

When I asked if her marriage had always been this unhappy, her response was no, that in the early years they had a good marriage "but then when my mother died, it seemed like I never recovered. I lost my spark, and it never returned. I lost interest in my children and John. Nothing seemed to matter anymore. At first, I felt sorry for John because I knew I was not being a wife to him. But then after his angry words, I figured he didn't deserve a wife, and I cared even less. Nothing matters anymore. I really wish I could die. It would be better for me and my family."

"How would you describe your feelings?" I continued.

"I have no energy," she said. "I have no interest in anything. I just try to sleep as much as I can."

"Do you feel angry toward John?" I inquired.

"No. I don't feel anything toward John," she said.

"Have you ever talked with your medical doctor about your feelings and your lack of energy?" I inquired.

"Right after Mother died, I went to see him once. He told me that I was depressed, and he gave me some antidepression pills. I took two or three of them, and they made me dizzy so I didn't take anymore."

"Did you go back to see the doctor?" I asked.

"No," she said. "I didn't want to tell him that I hadn't taken the pills he had prescribed."

"Have you ever known anyone who suffered from depression?" I asked.

"Not really," she said. "My mother told me about my grandmother and said that she died from depression after her son, my mother's brother, was killed in the war. But I never knew my grandmother."

"Do you think that all people who suffer from depression die from depression?" I asked.

"I don't know," Debbie responded.

"I've known lots of people who have suffered from depression," I said. "And none of them died. In fact, they are no longer suffering from depression. They are living happy lives." I went on to give Debbie a summary of depression, its symptoms, its causes, and its cures. I asked her if she thought she was depressed.

"I know I am depressed," she said. "I just don't know what to do about it. I'm not sure I can do anything about it."

"Sometimes when we have been depressed for a long time," I

said, "we get the feeling of hopelessness and we think that we will never get better. But I want you to know that depression can be healed. It takes some time, but when it is all over you can be happy again. You and John could have a good life together, and you could be the mother you always wanted to be. I have a good friend who specializes in helping people overcome depression. If I could set up an appointment with her, would you be willing to meet with her for a few weeks and let her help you walk through the valley of your depression and walk out to the mountain on the other side, where the sun is shining and the flowers are blooming?"

"I don't know if I have the energy, Dr. Chapman."

"I understand," I said. "But would you be willing to try?"

"I guess so," she said. (Most people who are deeply depressed are not highly motivated to enter counseling. Acquiescence is about as much as you can expect.)

"All right," I said. "I will set up an appointment for you and have her office call you. After you have met with her six times, I want to see you again and find out how you are doing." Debbie agreed and she left my office as slowly as she had entered.

The next week I saw John and recounted my time with Debbie and the strategy I had suggested to get her on the path to treatment. I asked him to be as positive as he could with Debbie, and I gave him the following list of "dos and don'ts" in his efforts to help her. If you or someone you know is married to a depressed husband or wife, I recommend this same list to you.

Don'ts

1. Don't tell her that she has nothing to be depressed about.
2. Don't tell her that everything is going to be OK.
3. Don't tell her to "snap out of it" or "pull yourself together."
4. Don't tell her that the problem is a spiritual problem.
5. Don't tell her that the problem stems from her family.
6. Don't tell her why you think she is depressed.
7. Don't give advice; rather, encourage her to listen to her counselor.

Dos

1. Do tell her that you are glad that she is going for counseling.
2. Do let her know that if she wants to talk, you want to listen.
3. Do receive her feelings without condemning them. If she says, "I'm feeling empty," your response might be, "Would you like to tell me about it?"
4. Do continue to take care of the children and things around the house.
5. Do look for life-threatening symptoms (suicidal talk or actions).
6. Do inform her counselor of such talk.
7. Do tell her that you believe in her and that you know she will come out of this.
8. Do encourage her to make decisions but don't force her.

"Remember, you can encourage her, you can be supportive, you can create a climate for her healing," I told John, "but you cannot be her therapist." I agreed to see John periodically while Debbie was in counseling and agreed that when her counselor recommended, I would begin marriage counseling with them.

The Treatment for Debbie

When I saw Debbie after her first six appointments with the counselor, there was a noticeable difference. She sat up straighter in the chair, she looked at me more frequently. Her face was not as forlorn, and she had gained a few pounds. Her major question for me was "What about taking medication?" The counselor had asked that she see a psychiatrist for an evaluation and perhaps take some medication. Debbie was reluctant to do this. I encouraged her to follow the advice of her counselor. I assured her that the counselor had worked with many other depressed people and that if she thought there might be a biological aspect to Debbie's depression, it was worth checking out. I reminded her that if the depression did have some biological basis, that medication could be extremely helpful. (I assured her that antidepressive medication is not addictive and that taking the medication was not a sign of weakness but of wisdom.

Eight months later when I began to do marriage counseling with John and Debbie, with Debbie's permission her counselor shared with me that although Debbie's depression seemed to be stimulated by her mother's death, it was really rooted in the fact that her father had sexually abused her as a child. Her mother's death had brought all these feelings to surface, and these plunged her into depression. The depression went untreated for almost a year and affected Debbie physiologically. Thus at that point, the medication was a necessary part of the treatment process. It was obvious to me at this juncture that Debbie had made tremendous progress. She was smiling, even joking at times. She was no longer spending her days in bed but was actively preparing meals, vacuuming floors, and doing other household tasks. She was attending church again. She was going shopping with her children, and she and John were going out to eat on a regular basis.

After approximately six to seven months of marriage counseling, I released John and Debbie. That was five years ago. Today, they have a healthy marriage, are actively involved with their extended family, have become leaders in the church, and are presently attending a class to develop their parenting skills.

John and Debbie's case illustrates that the causes of depression are not always readily discerned. Neither the individual who is depressed nor the spouse is likely to fully understand the source of one's depression. We can handle the normal depressions that last for a day or a week, but when depression persists and begins to affect our daily behavior, it is time to reach out for treatment.

GRIEVING OVER LOSS

At the heart of any treatment program for situational depression is helping the person walk through the grief process. Almost always situational depressions center around the loss of something, whether it be job, parent, child, integrity, or the loss of a dream. If the person is not allowed to grieve over the loss, he or she will almost always end up depressed. Mary's husband, Bill, went into a depression almost immediately after his father's death. Fortunately, Mary had just finished reading a book on depression in an effort to help a friend of hers. She recognized the symptoms of depression and realized that depression often follows a significant loss. She also realized that the process of grieving is facilitated by talking about the loss. So she started asking Bill questions about his father, more questions than she had ever asked in her life, and Bill started talking.

She learned of Bill's positive memories of going with his father on fishing trips in his childhood and adolescence. She also learned of painful memories that Bill had of his father's harsh discipline. She continued to ask questions and Bill continued to talk. She knew that she was helping him work through his grief and walk out of depression.

At first Bill was reluctant to talk about his father. He made such comments as "He's gone. There's no need to talk about him." But Mary would not be brushed off. She knew that Bill needed to talk and she wanted to listen. She realized that Bill's loss was not simply the death of his father but that his father's death had touched varied pain from his childhood—memories of Pop Warner football where his father was not on the sidelines to cheer; memories of his father's harsh words, but no memory of his father saying the words "I love you." She learned of Bill's good memories of his father providing for him, but also of the lurking fear that his father really did not care for him. Now all of these losses could never be replaced. Bill had never shared these thoughts and feelings with anyone, but Mary had the wisdom to pull them out and to listen sympathetically without trying to heal the wound herself.

Mary said such things as, "I can see how that would have been painful; how did you handle it at the time?" She stayed away from such condemning statements as "That was such a little thing; why did that bother you?" She listened and affirmed. She let Bill grieve. She helped him grieve.

In the first six months after Bill's father died, they had several of these conversations. Then every three months, she would bring up Bill's father again. For two years, she followed this process. At the end of two years, Bill's grief work was done and he was able to move on with life. He never entered a deep depression because he was allowed to grieve his losses. However, if Mary had not been there, there is the strong possibility that Bill would have gone into a deep and long depression after his father's death. That could have required extensive therapy for healing. Helping people grieve, by talking about their losses, is preventive medicine. It often averts a serious depression.

BEING PREPARED

The wise spouse will make time to gain information on depression and grief. Sooner or later, we will all experience losses in life. These losses can lead us to healthy grief or unhealthy depression. The spouse who understands depression and the process of grief can be extremely helpful in these times of crisis. The spouse who does not understand the process can actually compound the suffering of his or her mate. Numerous books and articles are available in any public library on both the subject of grief and depression. The wise spouse will be informed and ready to help facilitate the process of grief and to ward off depression.

Let me summarize some of the key elements in helping a depressed spouse. Seriously depressed people will seldom take initiative to help themselves. They are overwhelmed with the darkness of life. Their constant companion is a sense of helplessness. Therefore, *be a caring spouse,* showing compassion and being encouraging. The role of the caring spouse is extremely important. If the depression lingers more than a few weeks, encourage the spouse to talk with a counselor, minister, or a physician. If such encouragement goes unheeded, then tell your spouse that you are going for help, that you cannot sit idly by and watch him/her suffer.

My suggestion is that you *contact a counselor or minister and express your concern about your spouse* and how his depression is affecting you. *Ask the counselor for recommended readings and advice on how you can be helpful to your spouse.* Learn everything you can about depression. Review the "Dos and Don'ts" on pages 203–204.

Hopefully, your efforts to be a positive change agent will serve to motivate your spouse to reach out for professional help. Whatever the source of depression, there is always hope if the depressed person can get appropriate physical, psychological, or spiritual help.

EPILOGUE

It will be obvious by now that this is not a book for casual reading. It is a book to be pondered. The issues discussed have enormous consequences upon marriage and family in particular and upon society at large. Most importantly, this book calls for action. It is my hope that the passive reader who's in a troubling marriage will be jolted to reality and take steps that hold the potential of creating positive change in the marriage.

The people you have met in these pages may not have described your situation perfectly, but they are close enough that you have identified with their pain. More importantly, their stories have stimulated a fresh awareness of your own pain. It is not my intention to leave you wallowing in your pain but rather to challenge you to take a fresh look at your marriage. I understand that this may be difficult, especially if you have lived in a troubled marriage for a long time. At least you have the advantage of knowing that time alone does not heal the troublesome behaviors that we have described in this book. Perhaps this knowledge will encourage you to take a new approach.

One common response to a troubling marriage is to withdraw and not deal with the problem. The person withdraws from the spouse, the children, sometimes even from life, hoping the problem will go away. The person pulls the covers over her head and goes into hibernation, and depression often follows. This approach simply compounds the problem. Someone must now care for the children and eventually care for you. This withdrawing behavior makes things worse instead of better.

Another form of this is to take the kids, get out of the house and never return. While a temporary separation may be helpful in such a situation, a prolonged separation creates numerous other problems. It is in fact a method of withdrawal and denial and refusal to deal with the real issues in the marriage. This is not a constructive approach to the problem. Instead of withdrawing, our need is for action—for definite, loving solutions. Those solutions, based on reality living, can work.

The journey toward becoming a positive change agent in your marriage begins by saying no to the commonly held myths discussed in chapter 3. As long as you are held in bondage by these myths, you will never be able to take the positive steps of reality living. Let me review those myths and ask you to answer two questions: 1. Have I believed these myths in the past? 2. Will I continue to believe these myths in the future? If your answer to the first question is "yes," I hope your answer to the second question will be "no."

Here are the myths:

1. *My state of mind is determined by my environment.* Have you fallen into the trap of believing that your happiness is determined by your spouse's behavior?

2. *People cannot change.* Have you allowed yourself to become discouraged by believing that your spouse will never change his/her troublesome behavior?

3. *When you are in a bad marriage, there are only two options—resign yourself to a life of misery or get out.* Have you allowed yourself to be sidetracked by becoming obsessed with the question, "How can I get out of this marriage and get on with my life?" Or, have you been sidetracked by yielding to the conclusion that "My life is miserable, but there's nothing I can do about it"? Neither of these sidetracks

will lead you to the terminal of an intimate marriage.

4. *Some situations are hopeless.* Have you also concluded that your situation falls into this category—hopeless? To believe this myth is to underestimate the power of your own potential. It creates a defeatist attitude that stifles positive motivation.

Perhaps you have believed one or more of these myths in the past. I hope that the stories in this book have helped you understand that these myths are untrue. Your environment does not determine your happiness. Your spouse's behavior cannot keep you from living a happy, fulfilled life. People can change and often do when properly motivated. A person in a bad marriage has more than the two options of divorce or misery. You can become a positive change agent in a troubled marriage. No situation is hopeless. Because we are human, we have the capacity for change. When we change the way we think and behave, the situation changes. Yes, there is hope for even the most troubled marriage.

Refusing to believe these commonly held myths prepares you to become a positive change agent in your marriage by applying the principles of reality living. Let me review these principles.

Reality Number One: I am responsible for my own attitude. This reality affirms that I am responsible for my own state of mind. Attitude has to do with the way I choose to think about things. This reality allows you to refuse to believe the myths we have discussed above. We choose what we will believe. You can believe that your marriage is hopeless, or you can believe "there has got to be a way to turn this marriage in a positive direction." Each of us chooses his or her own attitudes.

Reality Number Two: Attitude affects actions. The reason attitudes are so important is that they affect our actions. By actions, I mean our behavior and words. If we have a pessimistic, defeatist, negative attitude, it will be expressed in negative words and behavior. If we choose to think optimistically, it will show up in our words and behavior. You may not be able to control your environment, but you can control the way you think about your environment, and your attitude will affect your behavior.

Reality Number Three: I cannot change others, but I can influence others. Most couples believe they cannot change their spouse, but they often overlook the fact that they can and do influence their spouse. Because we are relational creatures, we are all influenced by the words and behavior of those around us. We cannot force our spouses to change what we consider to be undesirable behavior, but by our words and our behavior we can influence them in a positive direction. All of society is built upon this reality. Exerting my influence upon my spouse has tremendous potential for stimulating positive change.

Reality Number Four: My actions are not controlled by my emotions. Emotions are the spontaneous feelings we experience as we encounter life. However, man is more than emotions. Emotions stimulate us to take action, but our emotions must be tempered by our thoughts and our desires. Otherwise, negative emotions would always lead to negative actions. If, however, I acknowledge that I am angry about my spouse's behavior but I have a desire to build an intimate marriage, I conclude that I will first ask, "What motivated my spouse to the behavior that made me angry? What is going on inside of him, and what would be my most productive response to his behavior?" Tempering emotions with my thoughts and desires will more likely lead me to take constructive actions. My actions need not be controlled by my emotions.

Reality Number Five: Admitting my imperfections does not mean that I am a failure. None of us is perfect. You may have concluded that the major problem in your marriage is your spouse's troublesome behavior. Even if this is true, it does not mean that your behavior is above reproach. Often, the first step in becoming a positive change agent is to acknowledge that your own behavior in the past has been inappropriate. Acknowledging this to yourself and your spouse may prepare the way for a more positive approach in the future. Admitting your own imperfections does not mean that you bear all the responsibility for your troubled marriage. It simply means that you are willing to accept responsibility for your own improper actions. Taking such responsibility does not mean that you are a failure, but rather it is a sign of maturity.

Reality Number Six: Love is the most powerful weapon for good in the world. Meeting your spouse's emotional need for love has the greatest potential for stimulating positive change in his/her behavior.

Since love is our deepest emotional need, the person who meets that need will have the greatest influence on our lives. Perhaps in the past you have not been loving in your words and behavior toward your spouse. Most likely this is because your spouse's behavior has not stimulated warm loving feelings toward him/her. Thus, you must return to Reality Four and realize that your actions need not be controlled by your emotions. You can love your spouse even though you may not have warm feelings toward him/her.

Remember, love is not essentially a feeling; it is a way of thinking and behaving. Love is the attitude that says, "I choose to look out for your interests. How may I help you?" This attitude will lead to loving actions. Such actions, in turn, meet the emotional need for love in your spouse and stimulate positive emotions inside, making it easier for him/her to reciprocate your love. Understanding the primary love language of your spouse will make this process much more effective.

If kind and tender loving acts do not produce positive change, then perhaps it is time for kind yet firm tough love. We have shared many examples of tough love in the preceding chapters. Remember, tough love is no less love. In fact, it may be the only kind of love your spouse can receive. It may be even more difficult than tender love. In expressing such tough love, you may have to go against the emotion of fear of what your spouse will do when you take such loving action. Again, Reality Number Four reminds us that our actions need not be controlled by our emotions. Love asks the question, "What is the best thing I can do for my spouse?" Tender or tough, love is the most powerful weapon for good in the world.

Applying the six principles of reality living to your marriage may be the most difficult thing you have ever done, but I can assure you that it holds the greatest potential for the well-being of your marriage. Reality living refuses to believe that your situation is hopeless. It chooses, rather, to believe in the power of human potential for change and recognizes that all of us are influenced daily by those who are part of our lives. The more intimate the relationship, the greater the influence. Thus, the marriage relationship holds tremendous potential for influencing a spouse to make positive changes. The key is in learning how best to exert this influence.

I sincerely hope that this book will help guide you toward becoming an effective, positive change agent in your marriage.

In applying the principles of this book, you may well need the help and encouragement of a friend, minister, or counselor. It is always a sign of maturity to reach out for help. We were not made to live in isolation. We reach our highest potential when we work together in community. You may wish to share this book with your counselor and let him/her help you apply these reality principles to your life and marriage.

If, in applying the principles of reality living to your marriage you experience significant growth, if you and your spouse overcome the troublesome barriers which we have discussed in this book, please share your story with others. Telling your story may encourage others in a troubled marriage to reach out for help. If we can all be more open about our own marital struggles and the steps we are taking to stimulate positive change, we can create a climate of hope which is desperately needed in modern society. If you share your story and I share my story, together we can make a difference in the world.

If you are interested in information about other books written from a biblical perspective, please write to the following address:

Northfield Publishing
215 West Locust Street
Chicago, IL 60610